AN INTRODUCTION T

The Ashgate World Philosophies Series responds to the remarkable growth of interest among English-language readers in recent years in philosophical traditions outside those of 'the West'. The traditions of Indian, Chinese, and Japanese thought, as well as those of the Islamic world, Latin America, Africa, Aboriginal Australian, Pacific and American Indian peoples, are all attracting lively attention from professional philosophers and students alike, and this new Ashgate series provides introductions to these traditions as well as in-depth research into central issues and themes within those traditions. The series is particularly designed for readers whose interests are not adequately addressed by general surveys of 'World Philosophy', and it includes accessible, yet research-led, texts for wider readership and upper-level student use, as well as research monographs. The series embraces a wide variety of titles ranging from introductions on particular world philosophies and informed surveys of the philosophical contributions of geographical regions, to in-depth discussion of a theme, topic, problem or movement and critical appraisals of individual thinkers or schools of thinkers.

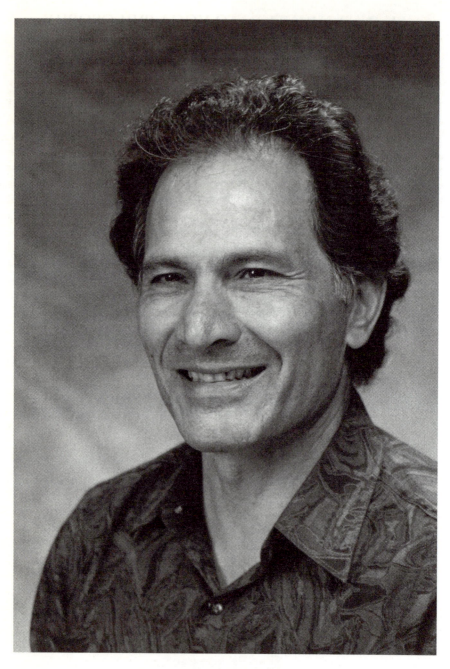

Dr Ashok Kumar Malhotra
SUNY at Oneonta

An Introduction to Yoga Philosophy

An annotated translation of the Yoga Sutras

ASHOK KUMAR MALHOTRA
SUNY at Oneonta

Ashgate
Aldershot • Burlington USA • Singapore • Sydney

© Ashok Kumar Malhotra 2001

All rights reserved. No part of this publication may be reproduced, stored in a retrieval system, or transmitted in any form or by any means, electronic, mechanical, photocopying, recording, or otherwise without the prior permission of the publisher.

Published by
Ashgate Publishing Limited
Gower House, Croft Road
Aldershot, Hants
GU11 3HR
England

Ashgate Publishing Company
131 Main Street
Burlington
VT 05401–5600
USA

Ashgate website: http://www.ashgate.com

The author has asserted his moral right under the Copyright, Designs and Patents Act, 1988, to be identified as the authors of this work.

British Library Cataloguing in Publication Data
Malhotra, Ashok Kumar, 1940–
   An introduction to yoga philosophy: an annotated translation of the Yoga Sutras. – (Ashgate world philosophy series).
   1. Patanjali–Yoga Sutras. 2. Yoga
   I. Title.
   181.4'52

US Library of Congress Cataloging in Publication Data
Patañjali.
   [Yogasutra. English.]
   An introduction to yoga philosophy: an annotated translation of the Yoga Sutras / Ashok Kumar Malhotra.
   p. cm. Includes bibliographical references.
   ISBN 0–7546–0524–8 (Hbk) – ISBN 0 7546 0564 7 (Pbk) (alk. paper)
   1. Yoga–Early works to 1800.   I. Malhotra, Ashok Kumar, 1940–.   II. Title.
   B132.Y6P313 2001
   181'.452–dc21

2001022060

ISBN 0 7546 0524 8 (Hbk)
ISBN 0 7546 0564 7 (Pbk)

This book is printed on acid free paper

Typeset in Times Roman by Manton Typesetters, Louth, Lincolnshire, UK.

Printed and bound in Great Britain by MPG Books Ltd, Bodmin, Cornwall.

To all those students of the State University of New York at Oneonta who have devotedly studied Yoga with me during the past twenty-five years and to Zach, a high school student, whose love for the Star Wars films inspired me to add the section on Yoga and Yoda

Contents

Preface viii

Part I The multidimensionality of Yoga

1 An interdisciplinary approach to understanding Yoga 3
2 Yoga as philosophy 6
3 Yoga as science 8
4 Yoga as psychology 10
5 The varieties of Yoga in the West 15
6 Patanjali: founder of the Yoga system 17
7 The four pillars of the *Yoga Sutras* 19

Part II A new rendition of the *Yoga Sutras* with commentary

8 *Samadhipada*: total mental stillness or tranquillity as the goal of Yoga 25
9 *Sadhanapada*: the method of Yoga 33
10 *Vibhutipada*: accomplishments of Yoga 42
11 *Kaivalyapada*: total liberation or salvation as the final goal 52

Part III Yoga and health

12 Yoga and healing: the medical connection 61
13 Practical aspects of Yoga 64

Part IV Yoga and Yoda

14 The *Star Wars* connection 89
15 Conclusions 101

Glossary 102
Bibliography 107
Index 108

Preface

Yoga has been with us for at least 2,500 years. As the present century opens with the dawning of the new millennium, Yoga's popularity has picked up speed as never before. People of all ages are drawn to it for reasons of physical health, mental contentment and spiritual enrichment. Yoga has stood the test of time because those who have indulged in it have received many beneficial results. It is an unusual system of physical and mental fitness, which benefits the person, without any harmful effects. Moreover, it is unique because its practice ranges from very simple to extremely complex exercises, which vitalize every aspect of the human body, mind and spirit. Its technique is available to anyone whether the individual is a supple child or an ageing adult. Since throughout the ages athletes, singers, artists, scientists, philosophers, actors, politicians, workers and even soldiers have benefited from its practice, it is no wonder that Yoga has earned a reputation as a holistic system whose goal is the perfection of the complete person.

Most people who are attracted to Yoga's promise of personal improvement and well-being are bogged down by its complexity and therefore settle for a superficial knowledge of it. Others, who have a genuine desire to unravel the mystery of the discipline, find that a vast majority of translations of the original text of the *Yoga Sutras* are either incomprehensible or written in a language that is incommensurate with the abilities of the present day reader. When I was growing up in India and studied the text under the tutelage of a guru, he presented its content to the class as if it were written for undergraduate students. The teacher made no attempt to suggest that there was anything esoteric about the substance of the text. Learning the *Yoga Sutras* in this fashion was an exciting venture.

For the past twenty years, while teaching Yoga to undergraduate classes in the United States, I have found that students are definitely excited to probe into the core content of the *Yoga Sutras*. What slows them down is the fear that since it is an old text, written in an ancient language and translated into incomprehensible English, it will be inaccessible to them. Though the desire to delve deeper into its content is there, the apprehension of not grasping its true meaning discourages the student from taking up the exhilarating challenge of studying the text. To bring back this excitement to the reading and comprehension of the *Yoga Sutras*, I have written this book in a language that captures the essential ideas of the text in words and phrases that are easily understood by undergraduate students as well as the general reader.

The format of the book is simple. The first part presents the multidimensional aspects of Yoga by locating its proper place among the disciplines of philosophy, science and psychology. It also includes the popular versions of Yoga in the West. The second part offers a new rendition of the text of the *Yoga Sutras* in a language that is straightforward and comprehensible to undergraduate students. Every effort is made not to use words and phrases which will hinder the smooth reading of the text. In this part, short commentaries are presented to highlight the meaning of various statements (*Sutras*). Rather than explain the significance of each statement (*Sutra*), commentaries are offered on groups of related statements (*Sutras*) because of their coverage of common themes. The third part of the book presents Yoga's connection to health by comparing Yoga's holistic view of healing with the limited perspective of medical science. Furthermore, this part describes the practical aspects of Yoga through a guided tour of physical, breathing, relaxation and meditation exercises. A number of basic exercises are described so that a student with or without any background in Yoga can practise them. The fourth part compares the basic ideas of Yoga, the epic *Ramayana* and the *Bhagavad Gita* to the underlying philosophy of the *Star Wars* films. It reveals parallels between the idea of consciousness and the force, the qualities of the Yogi and Yoda, and the rigorous training of Yoga students and Jedi Knights.

In writing this book, I have been guided by some of the major translations. I am thankful to the authors for their scholarly help. Dan Bristol, a 1999 SUNY Oneonta graduate and a friend, has helped improve the language of the entire text so that it will be suitable for undergraduate students as well as the general reader. He has also provided valuable editorial assistance without which this book would not be in its present form. Cindy Budka, currently attending SUNY Oneonta, deserves thanks for reading the entire manuscript and suggesting some crucial amendments. Marge Holling's generous spirit, as always, has worked wonders in putting the manuscript into its final form, ready for classroom use as well as for publication. Professors Douglas Shrader, David Cooper and Purusottama Bilimoria merit my heartfelt thanks for going over every page of the manuscript with a fine tooth comb. Finally, Sara Lloyd deserves thanks for consenting to publish this work. All photographs appear courtesy of James Belleau.

Ashok Malhotra
2 February 2001

Part I
The multidimensionality of Yoga

CHAPTER ONE

An interdisciplinary approach to understanding Yoga

The discipline of Yoga has enchanted readers and practitioners for centuries. It has more adherents now than ever before. What are the reasons for this enchantment and enthusiasm? Is it the mystique associated with the discipline, or the multi-sided content, or the step-by-step procedural practice that has drawn scholars, followers and curiosity seekers to it? Scholars have revealed their interest through the presentation of a multiplicity of interpretations; while followers make enthusiastic claims about the benefits accrued from its practice, curiosity seekers are attracted to it because of their expectation of an 'instant high'. Depending upon one's background and intentions, Yoga has something for everyone whether they are psychologists, philosophers, scientists, religionists or practitioners. As a body of knowledge about the mysterious nature of existence and a practical method to realize this wisdom here and now, Yoga offers an integral approach. In an artistically crafted system, Yoga brings together the disciplines of philosophy, psychology, science and religion. All of these fields are intertwined in the system of Yoga, providing unique yet related ways of unravelling the mystery of human existence. Since Yoga is one of the most ancient and enduring disciplines of India, it must be understood that we are engaging in a subject that is not just a philosophy or a psychology, but a *path* of salvation as well. In Yoga, philosophy, psychology and science come together to provide myriad ways to disclose the mystery of human existence.

Let us first analyse the literal meanings of philosophy, psychology, science and Yoga. The term 'philosophy' is derived from the words *philia* meaning love and *sophia* meaning wisdom. Philosophy, then, is the 'love of wisdom' or a continuous and spontaneous zest for intellectual inquiry. A philosopher is one who is deeply involved in critical inquiry about the justification of things, ideas and disciplines. Every discipline has a philosophical aspect, and it is the work of the philosopher to examine this feature. For example, when a psychiatrist becomes aware of the presuppositions of his discipline and brings them to the critical scrutiny of his intellect, he is no longer acting as psychiatrist but as philosopher. Similarly, when an artist starts actively wondering about art itself and asks herself about the nature, function and criticism of art, she has moved from the domain of art into the domain of philosophy. In the same way, it can be argued that historians, lawyers, mathematicians and other professionals reach a point in their respective disciplines where they cannot help becoming philosophers.

The term 'psychology' derives its meaning from the words *psyche* and *logos*. The history of the word *psyche* has been the history of our changing views of the human being. Originally, in Greek mythology, *psyche* was regarded as the personification of the soul, depicted as a young woman with butterfly wings, something that has everlasting enchantment, but cannot be grasped without disciplined effort. In religion, *psyche* became the soul and was regarded as a force separate from the body, which survived death. Later it came to be identified with the spirit, which as a life force guided the emotions and essential bodily movements. During the sixteenth century, it came to mean the mind or the thinking component of a human being. More recently, it has been identified with consciousness as distinguished from other facets of a human being such as body, sensing, perceiving and thinking. In the twentieth century, it was referred to as the personality or the self. From all these descriptions, we can deduce that *psyche* is the principle of consciousness, referred to as mind, soul, spirit or self. *Logos*, on the other hand, means reasoning, inquiry or discourse. Putting the two together, psychology becomes the study of consciousness or the self.

The word 'science' is derived from *scientia*, meaning knowledge. However, it is a special kind of knowledge, gained through the controlled observation of facts. It not only describes and explains facts, but offers predictions of their future behaviour as well. Its results are publicly shareable, linguistically expressible, quantitatively measurable and experimentally testable, that is its results can be expressed through ordinary language, measured through empirical instruments, conveyed through the tools of mathematics and logic, tested in a laboratory setting and replicated in another laboratory by another experimenter.

Before we can decide whether or not philosophy, psychology and science are suitable concepts to associate with Yoga, we must first specify the meaning of that term. The word Yoga is derived from the Sanskrit *yuj*, which has been variously interpreted by different scholars and thinkers. One of these meanings implies a union or an assimilation of two seemingly different entities. In this context, Yoga means the union of the essential self of a human being with the essence of the universe. This popular interpretation of Yoga suggests that the essential human spirit and the spirit of the universe are identical in nature. Human ignorance with respect to this essential fact results in the belief that a human being is separated from the essence of the universe. Yoga provides a method to realize this union between the human spirit and that of the universe.

The other meaning of *yuj* appears to be the direct opposite of the first because it implies a disunion of seemingly similar things. According to this interpretation, a human being is a combination of a material organism and pure consciousness. The everyday, 'average' existence, where each human being is trained and conditioned to accept and conform to arbitrary linguistic distinctions, social, cultural and scientific values as well as personal likes and dislikes, leads one to accept one's bodily and mental existence as the only reality. One thinks of consciousness as a by-product of biophysical processes. The aim of Yoga is to help each human being to break these artificial barriers of language, society and personal idiosyncrasy. Yoga provides a step-by-step procedure to dismantle the fetters of these conditioning elements so that the individual may realize the separate existence of one's reality, which is pure consciousness. Once the individual grasps that he is essentially pure consciousness different and separate from psychophysical processes, he is disunited from his false notions. At the same time the individual is also united in his thoughts, feelings, emotions and actions to his real self.

Since Yoga deals with consciousness in both its empirical and transcendental aspects, as well as in its intimate relationship to the self, it is clearly a system of psychology. Moreover, it also offers a step-by-step method through which one can perfect one's body and mind for enlightenment to take place here and now. Furthermore, the Yoga method can be used by anyone and its results can be replicated. Thus, it appears that Yoga is both a psychology and a science. Now a question can be raised, in what sense does philosophy enter into it? As pointed out earlier, each discipline, scientific or otherwise, has a philosophical aspect. When the theoretician, the teacher or the practitioner becomes self-reflective of her specific discipline and attempts to examine critically its assumptions, concepts and goals, at this point she becomes a philosopher. Similarly, underlying the psychological science of Yoga is the philosophical attitude that is involved in the definition, meaning, method and goals of Yoga. It not only examines the assumptions, concepts and aims of Yoga, but also provides a justification for them. Thus, we can say that in the Yoga system, philosophy, psychology and science are intertwined, and that they complement each other, embellishing the value of the discipline.

CHAPTER TWO

Yoga as philosophy

The systems of Yoga and Samkhya, which were created during the period 500–200 BC, have been studied together in the Indian philosophical tradition. One of the main reasons for this juxtaposition is the fact that the Samkhya philosophers offer a metaphysical view of reality, which is eagerly adopted by the Yoga system, whereas the Yoga thinkers provide a step-by-step method to achieve enlightenment, which is accepted by the Samkhya system. Since one offers a theory while the other a practical method, they complement each other and are studied as a complete system. Because Yoga borrows the Samkhya view of reality, it will be worthwhile to present a summary of the main points.

The Samkhya view of reality

According to the Samkhya thinkers, the universe consists of two separate realities: *Purusha* and *Prakriti*. *Purusha* is designated as pure consciousness whereas *Prakriti* is regarded as the unconscious material reality. As pure consciousness, *Purusha* is called a witness, a seer, an experiencer and an enjoyer of the artifacts of the material *Prakriti*. In contrast, as the unconscious material reality, *Prakriti* is the objective reality that is witnessed, seen, experienced and enjoyed by *Purusha*. Moreover, *Purusha* is considered to be immortal, spiritual and free, whereas *Prakriti* is regarded as mortal, material and determined.

The Samkhya thinkers hold that the interaction between the dialectically opposed realities of *Purusha* and *Prakriti* gives rise to all material and psychological forms in the universe. A human being is an interesting combination of these two contrary realities. As *Purusha*, a human being is pure consciousness or conscious self, and as *Prakriti,* a human being is a psychophysical self. The Samkhya thinkers assert that though a human being possesses a dual nature, his essential self is *Purusha* and not *Prakriti*. When we ignore the presence of pure consciousness (*Purusha*) in us and believe that our essence is nothing more than the psychophysical self (*Prakriti*), this leads to physical, mental and spiritual suffering. The mistaking of the immortal, spiritual and free for the mortal, material and determined is the main reason for this suffering. Thus, the goal of the Samkhya philosophy is to prepare the individual for discriminative knowledge, which is the realization that one's true nature is the immortal and free *Purusha* rather than the mortal and determined *Prakriti*. This discriminative knowledge equals enlightenment.

What is the reason for this mistaken identity? The Samkhya thinkers offer their theory of the evolution of the universe as an explanation for this confusion. In its unadulterated form, *Purusha* is pure consciousness. Similarly, in its primal form, *Prakriti* is a harmonious unity of three qualities of pleasure (*sattva*), pain (*rajasa*) and indifference (*tamasa*). Because of their close proximity, *Purusha* looks at *Prakriti*. This witnessing of *Purusha* upsets the balance of the three qualities in the heart of *Prakriti* and is responsible for starting the process of evolution.

  The first to arise are the three mental evolutes of intelligence (*buddhi*), ego-sense (*ahamkara*) and understanding (*manas*). The second to appear are the twenty physical evolutes, consisting of the five sense organs, the five motor organs, the five essences and the five elemental substances. In a human being, the three mental evolutes of intelligence, ego-sense and understanding make up the ordinary consciousness (*chitta*) whereas the twenty physical elements constitute the body. These twenty-three evolutes that make up the mind-body complex constitute the psychophysical self (*Prakriti*), whereas *Purusha* comprises the conscious self of a human being. According to Samkhya philosophers, since all consciousness belongs to *Purusha*, its activity of looking at the intelligence, ego-sense, understanding, five sense organs and five motor organs makes them conscious. Though these evolutes of *Prakriti* have only borrowed consciousness, they begin to believe that consciousness is their sole property rather than that of *Purusha*. This mistaken belief of the psychophysical self that it is the source of all conscious activity leads us to ignore the presence of *Purusha* within and to accept ourselves as nothing more than the mind-body complex. This conviction leads to a fall from the level of spiritual and free *Purusha* to that of material and determined *Prakriti*. According to the Samkhya system, this mistaken belief is at the heart of all human suffering. One can eradicate this misery through discriminative knowledge, which amounts to accepting one's real nature as *Purusha* as distinct from *Prakriti*. This discriminative knowledge is conducive to the blissful state of enlightenment.

  The Samkhya system suggests the path of *Gnana Yoga* or path of knowledge to achieve this discriminative knowledge. Since people have different abilities, this path is unsuitable for all those not possessing the required intellectual endowments. Furthermore, this path is too theoretical to appeal to a majority of people whose inclinations are pragmatic. In contrast, the Yoga system, which accepts the Samkhya metaphysics wholeheartedly, contributes its own practical method consisting of a step-by-step procedure to achieve the highly sought-after discriminative knowledge of one's real self (*Purusha*) as distinct from the psychophysical self (*Prakriti*).

CHAPTER THREE

Yoga as science

As mentioned earlier, the word 'science' refers to a specialized form of knowledge that is gained through observation and is tested by experience. Science utilizes the empirical method to describe and explain facts and offers predictions of their future behaviour. Its results can be verified and replicated by other researchers. Those who regard Yoga as science believe that the content, method and results of the system are empirically based and can be tested through experience. In their opinion, the Yoga masters were the first great scientists, who researched the inner world of human beings before any psychologist came to the scene. Their succinct description of levels of consciousness, clear explanation of the causes of affliction and a step-by-step procedure to eliminate suffering are clear indications of Yoga being a science.

Yoga compares the mind to a stormy ocean, which is agitated by sensations, perception, emotions, images, ideas and values. Since we are taught to identify ourselves with the state of our mind, we become whatever our mind is sensing, feeling, imagining or thinking at any moment. Because our mind is constantly bombarded by information, originating from internal or external sources over which we have no control, it is in a state of restlessness. The condition of our mind colours our view of what we are. If we are feeling agitated or morose, stressful or helpless, happy or sad, we identify ourselves with this particular state of the mind. Since a great part of our life is spent believing that we are nothing more than this tiny agitation in the ocean of our mind, we forget our real nature to be pure and restful consciousness.

One of the principal goals of Yoga is to help the individual take control of oneself and one's destiny. Its aim is nothing less than the mastery of the entire person through the formation of good habits of the body, heart and mind. In order to achieve this perfection, Yoga offers a step-by-step procedure called the *Ashtanga Yoga*. This method consists of eight steps, which are arranged in a hierarchical order:

1 *Yamas* (five restraints)
2 *Niyamas* (five disciplines)
3 *Asanas* (physical postures)
4 *Pranayama* (regulation of the vital force)
5 *Pratyahara* (sense organ withdrawal)
6 *Dharana* (concentration)
7 *Dhyana* (meditation)
8 *Samadhi* (absorption)

The first five are called the external steps because they aim to help the individual to gain control of one's attitudes, body, breathing, emotions and sense organs. The last three are called the internal steps because they assist the individual to take charge of all mental modifications arising from inner or outer sources. *Yama* and *niyama*, involving ten principles of physical, moral and spiritual hygiene, help the individual to develop proper mental attitudes in order to be prepared for the difficult task of mastering one's body and emotions through the next two steps of physical postures (*asanas*) and regulation of life force (*pranayama*). By perfecting these four steps, when the student of Yoga is able to develop positive habits, she is ready to undertake the next step of sense withdrawal (*pratyahara*). Though the body, emotions and breathing are brought under control, the practitioner of Yoga is still receiving impressions of the external world through the five sense organs. By withdrawing the mind from the sense organs and by directing it towards the inner self, the student is able to cut off contact with the external world. Once this complete withdrawal of the senses has taken place, the individual is ready for the three internal steps of meditation.

The meditative steps of concentration (*dharana*), meditation (*dhyana*) and absorption (*samadhi*) take inventory of the inner world and work on the elimination of all sensations, perceptions, images, emotions, thoughts and values. By cleansing the mind of these superfluous contents, the student of Yoga takes control of the state of her mind by distinguishing the mind from the real self.* As the student masters the meditative steps, she wipes the mind clean of all contents. When the mind becomes free of these mental modifications, it sparkles like a clear crystal, which readily reflects the light of pure consciousness of one's real self. Once the individual achieves this state, she lives in the world, takes delight in its wonders, but remains detached from its attractions and allurements. This state is designated variously as that of bliss or happiness; of sorrowlessness or fulfillment; of salvation or total freedom.

* The how of shifting consciousness from the Ahamkara to the Mahat.

— 8 limbs: Ashtanga Yoga

CHAPTER FOUR

Yoga as psychology

In the ancient Hindu tradition, scholars followed the 'great sayings' style. It consisted of choosing an important word or a phrase or a significant statement from the philosophical or religious text around which the entire commentary was written. This system was used in the writing of commentaries on the *Bhagavad Gita* as well as the *Yoga Sutras*. Since the system of Yoga has many such words and statements we will pick *Sutra* number 2 from Part I of the *Yoga Sutras* and reveal its importance.

In the second *Sutra*, Patanjali tells us that Yoga is *chitta vritti nirodha*, meaning that Yoga is the total control or elimination of all mental fluctuations. The *chitta-vrittis*, or mental fluctuations, are five in number: right knowledge, wrong knowledge, fantasy, memory and sleep. These five constitute all the knowledge, beliefs, attitudes and ideas we have accumulated through the use of sense organs and intelligence. Thus all our sense-intellectual knowledge is placed in the category of *chitta-vrittis*. Such knowledge is useful in that it prolongs our physical existence, but it is limited. It only partially manifests the real self or consciousness, which lies buried in the centre of our being. In order to manifest and experience the real self or *sat chit ananda* (infinite existence, consciousness and joy), these mental modifications must first be checked, then controlled, then inhibited and finally transcended.

To transcend this ordinary knowledge is an extremely difficult task. Only a few devoted students will ever reach this ultimate goal of self-realization. Every one of us, in moments of solitude, has to some degree aspired to this kind of knowledge. During those rare moments, we are ready to give up anything to attain this *sat chit ananda* or self-realization. When we come out of our solitude and are surrounded by others, we drown this desire for self-understanding in the world of gossip, animal concerns, social norms and personal prejudices. The ultimate goal of self-realization, which lies buried under the daily chores of personal, social and national life, can be unearthed by following a strict method of discipline. Patanjali recognizes different levels of people's aspiration. Not everyone aspires to self-realization. People differ from one another in terms of their physical and psychological make-up, and so their desire for self-perfection and self-actualization must also differ. To accommodate the enormous diversity among human beings, Patanjali recommends different levels of realizing one's innermost self.

Patanjali accepts the Samkhya view of human nature. According to the Samkhya philosophy, our psychophysical organism consists of three *gunas* or components, which are *sattva, rajasa* and *tamasa*. *Sattva* means light or bright, and its predominance in an individual inclines him or her towards contemplation or meditation. Such a person is most contented and happy in intellectual pursuits. *Rajasa* means action or activity. Its predominance in a person predisposes one towards action, and such an individual is aggressive, passionate, courageous or, in short, a person of action. *Tamasa* means inertia, immobility and heaviness. Its predominance in an individual is expressed through physical and intellectual laziness. Such a person is incapable of initiating any physical or intellectual action. He or she is merely a follower or a devotee.

According to the Samkhya philosophy, all human beings are composed of these three *gunas* or qualities. The excess of any one of these qualities determines our psychophysical nature. Some of us are meditative, others active, and some are lazy most of the time. It may appear that our nature hinders us, and therefore it may not be equally easy for all of us to realize the pure consciousness that resides within us. Patanjali offers various ways through which each of us with our unique predispositions can obtain a glimpse into reality at our own pace. Using the Samkhya view of the human being, we can distinguish between three kinds of personalities:

1 The *sattvic* personality
2 The *rajasic* personality
3 The *tamasic* personality

The *sattvic* personality is inclined towards spiritual and intellectual activity; the *rajasic* is predisposed towards active, passionate and sensuous pursuits, whereas the *tamasic* person leans towards nothing in particular. However, for each of these personality types, there is a convenient method of self-realization. For the *tamasic* personality, there is *Bhakti Yoga*, or the path of devotion. For the *rajasic* person, there is *Karma Yoga*, or the path of action. For the *sattvic* personality, there is *Gnana Yoga*, or the path of knowledge. Let us examine each one of these personalities and their special paths in some detail.

The tamasic personality

First, there is the *tamasic* personality. Since this kind of person has a predominance of the quality of *tamasa*, he has no motivation to initiate a physical or mental action. Because this lack of initiative is a hindrance to the realization of the inmost self, he or she needs to be moved along the path by external forces, whether the motivation comes from a group, another individual or an image of a deity. The path of devotion fits such a person's needs. Since the *tamasic* person is burdened by and devoted to the values and beliefs of other people, he or she can find salvation in the company of others of similar beliefs and values.

In the path of *Bhakti Yoga*, the group experience and the shared belief in the personification of the deity are the guiding principles of self-realization. The intellectual and spiritual experience of the ultimate reality is minimized and brought down to the level of mere bodily experience. The focus of attention of the group is usually some physical representation of a personal god such as *Krishna* or *Shiva*. The personal god is loved as a father, mother, friend, child or beloved.

In terms of religious experience, the adoration of a deity is the ultimate preoccupation of the *tamasic* personality. A *tamasic* person takes the statue of the deity as the embodiment of its reality, and constantly chants the name of god during waking moments. The name of the deity is chanted loudly to dispel all thoughts, emotions and feelings that disturb the individual. Not only is the image of god appropriated through sense perception and chanting; it is also assimilated through bodily movements, group singing and dancing. By filling the sensual awareness with the image of god, by constantly chanting the name of god, and by blending the sound of the deity with bodily sensations, one feels lifted above the gross *chitta-vrittis* or psychophysical disturbances, and thus moves towards the underlying unity of one's real self. This method of *Bhakti Yoga* has been adopted and popularized by the Hare Krishna movement in America.

The rajasic personality

Second is the *rajasic* personality. Such a person has an abundance of *rajasa*. He or she is inclined towards action, passion and aggressiveness. A *rajasic* person is propelled by desires and emotions, and is constantly in pursuit of sensuous satisfaction or daredevil feats. Such a person is capable of initiating any action. He or she has both the physical equipment and the mental ability to go after the desired object. Since the *rajasic* person is out-going, externally oriented and indulges in excessive activity, such a person is restless, undergoes physical and mental exhaustion, and is extremely disturbed.

To become inwardly directed is a difficult task for the *rajasic* personality. However, there is a method, which can calm the nerves and reduce this restlessness. The method most suitable for the *rajasic* person is that of *Mantra Yoga*, which is part of *Karma Yoga*. The Sanskrit prefix *man* means to think or reflect, and *tra* means to eliminate disturbance. Thus, a mantra is an instrument that can eliminate disturbance when used as a means of reflection. Mantra also refers to a special sound, which can help the student to move from action to the source of action. The use of a mantra can also assist the active, passionate individual to sit down and withdraw his or her outwardly directed energies to their inner source.

Each mantra is a set of Sanskrit words corresponding to a certain mental vibration or level of consciousness. To change the focus of the outwardly directed personality, the mantra must first be chanted loudly. Once the practitioner finds it convenient and easy to focus the mind on the mantra, it should then be repeated silently. This meditative exercise will ultimately reveal the meaning of the mantra, and may lead to the realization of the deepest levels of consciousness, where all activity has its source.

There are many different mantras suitable for meditation, each related to a level of consciousness. The following mantras are those most frequently used:

1. *Sat chit ananda*: literally, 'infinite existence, consciousness and joy'. These three qualities make up the nature of ultimate reality. A spark of this reality resides in each human being as their essence.
2. *Tat tvam asi*: literally, 'you are that'. *Tat* refers to brahman, the objective universal reality, *twam* to atman, the subjective reality within each person, and *asi* to their identity. This mantra alludes to the identity between the human and universal essence.
3. *Neti neti*: literally, 'not this, not this'. This mantra is given to a meditator to caution him that the ultimate reality is beyond all descriptions. Even after one has the experience of it, the ultimate reality will defy characterizations. So 'neti neti' is the best way to describe this ineffable reality.
4. *Aham Brahman asmi*: literally, 'I am Brahman, the ultimate reality'. This mantra states that the essence of a human being is identical with that of the ultimate reality.
5. *Om*, the sound-symbol for the ultimate reality, contains within itself the secret to reach this reality. It is considered to be the highest mantra whose proper utterance can lead to illumination.

Om is regarded as the most significant of these mantras. There are various reasons for this. *Om* appears to be a word, but is not a word. Rather, it is a kind of symbol pointing to the ultimate reality. The sound *Om* is regarded as the creator, preserver and destroyer of all sounds. According to tradition, all the sounds in the cosmos come out of it, are sustained by it and ultimately merge back into it. It is the sound of ultimate reality. The vibration of the ultimate reality is contained within this sound and through it reality speaks to us. One who utters it loud and then silently will understand its meaning. If we think of the individual self as an aggregate of vibrations, then *Om* is the real focal point of that vibration, from which we are never disconnected. It is firmly believed in tradition that constant practice of this mantra brings restfulness, energy and a calm disposition. The Transcendental Meditation Movement has adopted a popularized form of the *Mantra Yoga*.

The sattvic personality

The *sattvic* person has a predominance of the *sattva* quality. Since the nature of this quality is joy and goodness, such a person is inclined towards spiritual, meditative and reflective pursuits. Because of this natural propensity, happiness is achieved by involving oneself in activities that cater to the development and expression of the intellect, mind and spirit. A *sattvic* person is capable of initiating and carrying out any intellectual or meditative action. He or she is more interested in revealing the secrets of the inner world by reading the holy books, philosophical works or lives of people who have had success in achieving enlightenment through their own efforts. Such an individual follows the path of *Gnana* or knowledge by reading books, interpreting them and imparting information to others. Their favourite places are libraries, forests or caves where they can feel that connection between themselves and the reality. Some of these individuals involve themselves in Yoga practice, while others become interpreters of scriptures or philosophical texts. Whatever course of action they might adopt, they are interested in obtaining their salvation through the path of knowledge or inward reflection. This path of *Gnana Yoga* is adopted by the followers of the Samkhya school of philosophy.

CHAPTER FIVE

The varieties of Yoga in the West

Yoga is one of the most ancient philosophical, psychological and scientific disciplines known. Although its earliest recorded origins date back between 500 and 200 BC, it still evokes the same awe, admiration and reverence from its serious followers as it did at the time of its inception. During its 2,500 year journey, the discipline of Yoga has been developed, changed, modified and, in the present day, converted into a fad. Yoga is so multi-faceted that it has something for everyone. In the West, Yoga has been understood in four different ways, each catering to the interests of people with varying dispositions. In his book *Superconscious Meditation* Dr Usharbudh Arya distinguishes between Hollywood Yoga, Harvard Yoga and Himalayan Yoga. To this scheme a fourth may be added – Cultic Yoga.

Hollywood Yoga, as its name suggests, caters to those whom popular slang describes as the 'beautiful people'. These are people who want merely to look young, stay young and feel young, both physically and mentally. They desire a slim figure, a young body and a long life. They want a discipline that can keep them physically fit and mentally alert, both regarded as assets in our youth-oriented culture. They look at Yoga from a special perspective to fulfil their special needs. For such people, Yoga is limited to a set of physical exercises to rejuvenate the skin, redden the cheeks, brighten the eyes and add curves to a flabby body. The form of Yoga that caters to these desires is the well-advertised *Hatha Yoga*. Anyone can practise it, provided that they are motivated and are willing to make time for the practice.

Harvard Yoga is more limited. It is the concern of scientists. The interest of scientists is not the performance of physical exercises in order to beautify the body and calm the mind, but rather to measure and study the effects of Yoga exercises on the human personality. Scientists wish to educate people, informing them of the influence of Yoga practice on the transformation of a human being. According to Dr Arya, these two perspectives are easily understood because they are closer to the mind whose orientation is materialistic, perceptual and technological. However, they are limited and superficial. The approaches of Hollywood Yoga and Harvard Yoga can sell a modified or watered-down product but cannot be mistaken for the real thing. The 'real Yoga' goes beyond both of these.

The third type, referred to as Cultic Yoga, is for the curiosity seekers, who are looking for an 'instant high'. In the West, these curiosity seekers practise a form of Yoga that has been modified to cater to their fashionable interests. In this popular version, emphasis is placed on the personal powers that have been achieved by the founders of certain religious and cultic groups. The leaders of these groups declare themselves to be in possession of enlightenment, which they can pass on to their disciples, through a word, a look or a touch. Disciples are told that they need no preparation or hard work to achieve this state of enlightenment, because the cult leader has the power to transmit it to anyone at will. This cultic form of Yoga has drawn a huge number of disciples to these charismatic leaders. Although the original Yoga system discusses many powers often claimed by cultists, it warns the disciple of their negative influence on achieving the ultimate goal of Yoga.

Himalayan Yoga is the true and authentic Yoga. Though it describes extraordinary powers gained through physical exercises, control of breathing and by the practice of meditation, Himalayan Yoga warns the serious student not to get attached to them. These accomplishments are regarded as obstacles to achieving the real goal of Yoga, which is total self-realization. Himalayan Yoga is based upon an ancient book, the *Yoga Sutras* of Patanjali. The text is divided into four parts. Part I deals with the meaning and goal of Yoga. Part II discusses the methods to achieve these goals. Part III describes the powers one may attain by following the strict discipline of Yoga. And Part IV delves into the ultimate goal of Yoga, which is total self-realization, also described as total liberation from all limitations of human existence.

CHAPTER SIX

Patanjali: founder of the Yoga system

Yoga first appeared as a system of philosophy between 500 and 200 BC. Its main ideas are presented in a text called the *Yoga Sutras,* composed by an Indian sage named Patanjali.

In Hinduism, there are 330 million gods and goddesses, of which the three most important ones make up the Hindu trinity. This trinity consists of *Brahma*, the Creator, *Vishnu*, the Preserver, and *Shiva*, the Destroyer. After *Brahma* creates the universe, the god *Vishnu* supports it. *Vishnu*, as the preserver, is seated in his heavenly abode upon a huge snake with many heads. The enormous body of this snake, which floats on the surface of an immense, cosmic ocean, acts as a comfortable bed for *Vishnu*. The snake represents time, and the ocean depicts the ever-changing universe in which we live.

There is an interesting story about Patanjali and how he created the Yoga system.[1]

> One day, as *Vishnu* was resting comfortably, the snake noticed that *Vishnu's* body began to shake and grow heavier. Afraid that he might be crushed, the snake said to *Vishnu*, 'You are shaking and your weight is increasing. Your weight is too much for me to carry. If you do not stop shaking, I will be crushed. Please tell me why this is happening.'
>
> *Vishnu* replied, 'I am watching the dance of *Shiva*, the god of destruction. His dance, even his very body, are both so entrancing that my entire body is caught up in his vibrations.'
>
> The snake asked, 'What does this vibration mean?'
>
> 'Since the secret of life and death is contained within the rhythmic vibrations of *Shiva's* dance, I could not help becoming caught up in it,' replied *Vishnu*.
>
> 'I have also felt this vibration and have learned a great deal from it. What I have learned from you and the vibration is the secret of life and death, the very meaning of life. Human beings desperately need this kind of knowledge. With your permission, I will go down to the world and impart this wisdom to them,' the snake implored.
>
> *Vishnu* agreed that the snake should go down and told him that human beings would need to put this wisdom into practice because possessing this secret would not be enough. The Preserver explained

---

[1] See B.K.S. Iyengar's *Light on the Yogasutras of Patanjali*, San Francisco: HarperCollins, 1993.

that in order to live a happy and contented life, human beings require three things: good speech, a healthy body, and a harmonious mind. Good speech comes from learning proper grammar. A healthy body comes from good posture and a proper diet. A harmonious mind is accomplished through cultivating proper mental discipline. *Vishnu* went on to explain that these three, taken together, could lead to enlightenment and even immortality.

So *Vishnu* instructed the snake to go down to earth and take birth as the son of a particular wise woman. This woman had prayed to *Vishnu* many times in order to be blessed with a child to whom she could impart her wisdom. The Preserver knew that this woman had already gained wisdom about the importance of good speech, a healthy body and a harmonious mind. He also knew that she would be willing to teach her wisdom to such an apt pupil as the snake, and so the snake was given permission to go to earth and be born as a human being.

Early one morning, as the wise woman was preparing for her prayer to the rising sun, she bent over to pick up some flowers. She held these flowers in her folded hands. As she opened her hands to offer the flowers to the rising sun, she beheld an extraordinary sight. A tiny snake crawled onto her open hands. When the woman and the snake made eye contact, the snake spoke to her.

'I have been sent by *Vishnu* to be your son,' the snake said. 'I would like to learn from you about the three things that human beings need in order to lead a happy and contented life on earth: grammar for good speech etc.'

The wise woman accepted him as her son and named him Patanjali. The name Patanjali is a compound of two words: *pata*, meaning a leaf, and *anjali*, referring to the gesture of folding hands in prayer.

Later in his life, Patanjali composed three major works. The first was a book on Sanskrit grammar, written around 500 BC. This work is considered to be the most perfect and authoritative text on grammar ever written. The second book, called the *Ayurveda,* dealt with health and ageing. It presented principles which, if put into practice, would free the body from disease and the rigours of age. The third book the *Yoga Sutras,* dealt with the physical, mental and spiritual exercises required to perfect the total person. Through physical postures different parts of the body can be perfected in order to defy the ageing process; through the breathing exercises, the emotions can be controlled; and through the meditative exercises, the mind can be disciplined. Utilizing the principles taught in the *Yoga Sutras* to create complete harmony in the body, emotions and the mind, the whole person can be perfected and the spark of divinity residing at the core of one's being can be realized.

CHAPTER SEVEN

The four pillars of the *Yoga Sutras*

The text of the *Yoga Sutras* is constructed in a unique way called the *sutra* style. This style of writing texts was developed in India because of the demands imposed by the Hindu oral transmission of teaching. The tradition required the student to commit all lessons to memory without writing them down. To facilitate this memorization process, teachers devised a unique system of condensing an entire text into a few statements called *Sutras*. Literally, a *Sutra* means a rope or a thread. Metaphorically, it can be called 'a garland of ideas' or 'a necklace containing pearls of wisdom'. Philosophically, a *Sutra* means a statement or an aphorism, which holds within itself the essential elements or quintessence of a theory. In the crafting of a *Sutra*, words were carefully chosen to convey a part of or the entire philosophical, psychological, scientific or religious doctrine. Patanjali, who adopted this style, conveys the essential knowledge of the entire system of Yoga through 196 aphorisms or *Sutras*.

These 196 *Sutras* are presented in the four parts of the text called the *Yoga Sutras*. Patanjali further condenses the entire text by highlighting the four focal points around which the entire system of Yoga revolves. The title of each part guides the student to pay full attention to the four pillars on which the wisdom of Yoga rests. These four parts of the *Yoga Sutras* are:

1   *Samadhipada*
2   *Sadhanapada*
3   *Vibhutipada*
4   *Kaivalyapada*

Samadhipada

Part I, called the *Samadhipada*, consists of 51 *Sutras*. As the title suggests, it focuses on the nature of *samadhi*. This part opens with the statement, 'Here now begins the study of Yoga' and closes with the statement, 'When the impressions of truth bearing wisdom are also destroyed, then the seedless trance (*nirbija samadhi*) arises.' The first statement makes it clear that this is a book on Yoga and not on another system. Moreover, this statement also implies that the reader is committing himself to this very important discipline. The last *Sutra* is plainly saying that when the practice of Yoga is undertaken seriously, one will be rewarded with *nirbija samadhi*, which means that all fluctuations of the mind will be stilled and there will be no seeds of disturbance left as residues. In the remaining *Sutras*, Patanjali describes the meaning and goal of Yoga; impediments to the attainment of trance (*samadhi*); practice and non-attachment as preliminary steps needed to remove these impediments as well as the roles of mantra and chant in the realization of trance.

Sadhanapada

Part II, called the *Sadhanapada*, consists of 55 *Sutras*. Its main concern is with *Sadhana* or the practice of the Yoga discipline. Practice consists of methods to achieve the goals of Yoga. Two main methods are discussed in this part. The first, called *Kriya Yoga*, is a preparatory method, which consists of three steps of austerity, introspection and ego surrender. The perfection of these steps will lead towards removing such psychological and spiritual blemishes as ignorance of reality, egotistical impulses, attachment, repulsion, clinging to life or fear of death. Once this preliminary practice is mastered, one can proceed to the main method called the *Ashtanga Yoga*. It consists of eight steps, which help the student to bring harmonious perfection in the physical, mental and spiritual aspects of one's being. Since this method aims at the crafting of a totally integrated person which will lead one to enlightenment, it is meant only for the serious aspirant.

Vibhutipada

This is the longest part consisting of 56 *Sutras*. Though it deals with powers achieved through Yoga exercises, it starts with a description of the meditative steps and ends with a depiction of total enlightenment through the illuminative consciousness. The first three *Sutras* describe the meditative steps of concentration (*dharana*), meditation (*dhyana*) and absorption (*samadhi*). These three constitute the internal steps that make possible the control of the mind. The remaining *Sutras* describe various powers achieved when concentration is directed towards different parts of the body, the mind and the universe. Ultimately, through making the mind one-pointed, a person can achieve many extraordinary powers, which are not usually available to an ordinary human being.

Kaivalyapada

This is the shortest of the four parts and comprises only 34 *Sutras*. It opens with the assertion that these extraordinary powers can be achieved through birth, drugs, chanting of sacred words, austerity or meditation. Furthermore, it warns the student against getting attached to these accomplishments. It delves into the layers of consciousness and recommends the development of the powers of discrimination so that the student can ascertain the difference between the lower and higher reality. This part ends with a description of the nature of liberation or total freedom from all limitations, where consciousness comes back to its original source.

Part II
A new rendition of the *Yoga Sutras* with commentary

* Kabir's poem

CHAPTER EIGHT

Samadhipada: total mental stillness or tranquillity as the goal of Yoga

Part I, consisting of 51 *Sutras*, deals with the definition and the goal of Yoga, impediments to tranquillity and preliminary ways of achieving total mental stillness. Each *Sutra* is crafted with the help of selected words and phrases to convey essential elements of a philosophical theory. There are two sets of *Sutras* in the text. One group deals with themes that are crucial to the Yoga system whereas the other presents an explanation of the central ideas. To provide a clearer understanding of their meaning, I will comment on groups of related *Sutras*, which have either central or explanatory status.

Sutras

Preliminary goal of Yoga

1.1 Here now begins the study of Yoga.
1.2 Yoga is the stilling of all mental fluctuations.
1.3 When the fluctuations are completely silenced the seer experiences one's true self as a witness to the world.
1.4 When they are not stilled, an individual identifies one's true self with these mental fluctuations.

Commentary The first *Sutra* introduces the reader to the Yoga text by indicating that its focus will be on the study of Yoga and not any other subject. Furthermore, this *Sutra* has an aura of seriousness about it because it asserts that the study of Yoga begins now, at this moment, and in this space.

However, the second *Sutra* is at the core of the entire system because it presents the quintessence of Yoga by offering a preliminary definition as well as its goal. It captures the essential elements of Yoga through a masterfully crafted statement, '*Yoga chitta vritti nirodha*'. Here *Yoga* refers to the subject matter at hand; *chitta* to the ordinary mind or consciousness; *vritti* to fluctuations in the mind; and *nirodha* to discipline, control and elimination. Yoga then is defined as 'the disciplining, controlling and stilling of all mental fluctuations'. Furthermore, this *Sutra* offers a preliminary goal of Yoga by implying that the true self of an individual is radically different than the fluctuations in the ordinary mind or consciousness. This true self can only be realized when these fluctuations are brought to a standstill and the mind has become totally calm.

The third *Sutra* makes it clear that the stilling of the ordinary mind will reap two major benefits for the student of Yoga. First, the student will achieve tranquillity of the mind and second, while basking in this peaceful state, she will experience the true self as the pure witnessing consciousness taking delight in the workings of the world.

The fourth *Sutra* describes the mental state of all of us who have not yet silenced these fluctuations. Since we identify ourselves with these fluctuations, we keep on conducting our daily lives by believing that we are nothing more than our temporary pleasures, pains, anxieties, worries, wishes and desires.

Kinds of fluctuations

1.5   There are five types of fluctuations, which are both painful and not painful.
1.6   They are correct knowledge, error, fantasy, sleep and memory.
1.7   Correct knowledge comes from direct perception, inference and verbal authority.
1.8   Error is mistaking the unreal for the real.
1.9   Fantasy is imaginary knowledge where words do not correspond to any substantial reality.
1.10 Sleep is the awareness lacking mental content.
1.11 Memory is the recollection of a previously experienced image.

Commentary   In these seven *Sutras*, Patanjali is asserting that our knowledge is nothing more than fluctuations in the mind or consciousness. Human beings use five ways to collect information of the outer and the inner worlds. These are designated as correct knowledge, error, fantasy, sleep and memory. We obtain correct knowledge through our own sense experience and logical reasoning as well as from the words of informed people. We receive our erroneous knowledge from false perception or faulty reasoning, or some unreliable source. Furthermore, we make up knowledge through fantasy, where we may use words that do not correspond to any substantial reality. We may create an imaginary world and believe it to be real or true. For example, one might create an image of oneself that does not correspond to what one really is.

Patanjali mentions sleep and memory as two further sources of ordinary knowledge. Sleep, which includes the experiences of daydreams, night dreams and dreamless sleep, and memory, which comprises the experiences of the past, fill our ordinary mind with reveries, anxieties, fears and other unfulfilled desires. According to Patanjali, these five sources provide all knowledge in the form of fluctuations in the ordinary mind or consciousness. Since at some times these fluctuations are painful while at other times they are not painful, our identification with these states offers us the impression that we are nothing more than these fleeting disturbances.

Our daily lives are thus far removed from the experience of our true nature, which is to be totally tranquil and peaceful. In the next few *Sutras*, Patanjali offers ways of controlling these mental fluctuations.

Preliminary ways to still the mind

1.12   These fluctuations can be brought to rest through practice and non-attachment.
1.13   Practice is the continuous effort to control these fluctuations.
1.14   Practice becomes firmly established when undertaken devotedly and uninterruptedly for a long time.
1.15   Non-attachment is complete self-control and total detachment from craving objects.
1.16   The highest non-attachment, which is the cessation of desire for all artifacts of material reality, is achieved when one discriminates between the psychophysical self and the true self.

Commentary   Since the goal of Yoga is to make the ordinary mind totally still, Patanjali suggests practice (*abhyasa*) and non-attachment (*vairagya*) as the two preliminary ways to control these fluctuations. The Sanskrit word *abhyasa*, which is translated here as practice, means forming habits of the body, mind and spirit. It is comparable to building character. As the instilling of good habits requires uninterrupted devotion, practice also demands the fulfilment of similar conditions for its success in silencing all mental fluctuations. Furthermore, practice needs to be aided by non-attachment, which asks for nothing less than the negation of desire for appropriating the artifacts of material reality. The formation of the good habits of practice and non-attachment will lead to the dawning of discriminatory knowledge where the individual will be able to view his or her true self as different from all mental fluctuations.

Stillness of the mind or consciousness

1.17   Practice and non-attachment lead to the first level of stillness of the mind or consciousness called *samprajnata samadhi*. Here the mind is centred on reasoning, reflection, joy and the ego-sense.
1.18   In the next level of stillness, called *asamprajnata samadhi*, all except the dormant mental fluctuations are brought to rest.

Commentary   By forming the good habits of practice and non-attachment, the student of Yoga is able to transcend the influences of the external world and is led to the threshold of the inner world of consciousness. When there is no longer the sway of material objects, and the entire outer world is shut down, the student is ready to delve into the inner world of mental activities. Patanjali utilizes the term *samadhi* to capture the mystery of this inner universe. *Samadhi* has two interrelated meanings. First, it depicts the last step of the eight-tiered method that aims to bring the aspirant to the threshold of enlightenment. Second, the term is used to describe seven levels of contemplative consciousness during the inward journey towards self-realization. Each one of these levels of *samadhi*, also called contemplative consciousness, is a stage on the mystic's way to achieving enlightenment, where in the last one, the student is rewarded with the experience of one's true self.

These seven stages of contemplative consciousness are arranged in a hierarchical order ranging from the lowest to the deepest level of tranquillity. The first two are named *samprajnata* and *asamprajnata samadhis* and are described in *Sutras* 17 and 18, whereas the other five – *savitarka, nirvitarka, savicara, nirvicara* and *nirbija samadhis* – are discussed in *Sutras* 42 to 51.

By perfecting the habits of practice and non-attachment, the mind of the student becomes totally oblivious to external stimulation and is brought to the threshold of consciousness. This stage of contemplative consciousness is called *samprajnata samadhi*. Here the mental states of reasoning (*vitarka*), reflection (*vicara*), joy (*ananda*) and ego-sense (*asmita*) become the focal point of concentration. Contemplation of each one of these requires a unique mental activity. Reasoning (*vitarka*) is aimed at obtaining the complete knowledge of the material (gross) object. As the contemplative activity is initially directed towards the object, the mind concentrates on the intermingling of the three elements of the object, the instrument of perception and the perceiver. Through continuous indulgence in this mental activity, the student is able to grasp these three components as one. However, in reflection (*vicara*), the focus of contemplation is subtle objects such as the causes of objects as well as the ego-sense. In the joy (*ananda*) stage, contemplation fixes its intention on freedom from constraining fetters of the material qualities, which results in the experience of pure delight. In the fourth stage, the aspirant concentrates on the ego-sense (*asmita*) and realizes the true nature of the principle of individuation and its activity through which it falsely identifies one's psychophysical self with the true self. While the contemplative consciousness performs these four acts of concentration in the *samprajnata samadhi*, it realizes that they must be transcended. To reach deeper levels of consciousness, the student must leave behind all these mental states. This stage of concentration is called *asamprajnata samadhi*.

Various ways to achieve stillness

1.19 Some are born with physical and mental endowments and can achieve the stillness of the mind effortlessly.

1.20 Others can achieve it through faith, energy, memory, concentration and discernment.

1.21 Some gain immediate access to it because they pursue it with abundance of energy and intensity.

Samadhipada: *The Goal of Yoga*

1.22   The success in achieving this stage is proportionate to the aspirant's intensity of motivation.
1.23   Stillness of the mind can also be attained through devotion to the *Perfect Yogi* or *Ishwara*.
1.24   The *Perfect Yogi* is a unique being who is uncorrupted by desire, suffering and action.
1.25   The *Perfect Yogi* is the original source of all knowledge.
1.26   The *Perfect Yogi*, who is unbounded by time, is the foremost teacher of all sages.
1.27   The *Perfect Yogi* expresses itself through the sound *Om*.
1.28   The constant repetition of *Om* and concentration on this symbol are sure ways of grasping the nature of the *Perfect Yogi*.
1.29   All obstacles to the realization of the true inner self are removed through the practice of recitation and meditation.

Commentary   After presenting a discussion of the importance of practice and non-attachment in the achievement of stillness of the mind, Patanjali cites other factors such as natural endowments, personal drive and strength of motivation. Moreover, in *Sutra* 23, Patanjali introduces the idea of a *Perfect Yogi*. By imbibing this ideal, a student can easily achieve stillness of the mind. The *Perfect Yogi*, who is described as the Master of Yoga, is the source of all knowledge; is the first teacher; is uncorrupted by the desires and afflictions of the world; and can be understood through the sound-symbol *Om*. The chanting and contemplation of *Om* can also facilitate the understanding of both the essence of the *Perfect Yogi* and the true nature of the inner self.

The sound *Om* is an important symbol in the Indian philosophical tradition. It is believed that the ultimate reality (*Brahman*) revealed itself through the universal vibration of *Om*. All the sounds have come out of it, are sustained by it and merge back into it. It is the source of all speech and thinking because it contains within itself all the vowels and consonants. Furthermore, the entire universe of galaxies, stars, planets, animals and humans owe their origin to this sound. Moreover, since *Om* is compared to an arrow, which is aimed at the ultimate reality of *Brahman*, one should begin and end one's prayers with it. Since it is believed to be the beginning, middle and end of all sounds, *Om* is recommended as the best mantra for meditation. Because of the significance assigned to it in the tradition, Patanjali recommends *Om* as one of the important aids in achieving tranquillity.

Disturbances of consciousness and their elimination

1.30   The nine impediments that hinder the mind or consciousness from gaining tranquillity are disease, mental sluggishness, doubt, carelessness, physical laziness, uncontrolled sensual craving, delusion, lack of perseverance and instability.

30 The Yoga Sutras *with Commentary*

1.31 Consciousness is further distracted by pain, anguish, unsteadiness of the body and irregular breathing.
1.32 These distractions can be controlled through concentration on a single object.
1.33 Consciousness can achieve clarity and calmness through the cultivation of friendliness towards the happy, compassion towards the miserable, joy towards the virtuous and indifference towards the non-virtuous.
1.34 Consciousness can also be made tranquil through the control of exhalation and retention of breath.
1.35 Steadiness of consciousness can be accomplished further by concentrating on some super-physical power.
1.36 Consciousness can attain serenity through concentration on the natural mental state of sorrowlessness.
1.37 Focusing the mind on those who have achieved the state of peacefulness can still consciousness.
1.38 By reflecting on the states of dream and deep sleep, consciousness can attain equilibrium and equipoise.
1.39 Consciousness can also develop one-pointed attention by concentrating on an object closer to one's heart.
1.40 Established in steadfastness, consciousness develops mastery over the tiniest atom and infinite space.

Commentary In the first two *Sutras* of this group, Patanjali outlines both mental and physical impediments to tranquillity. Disease, mental sluggishness, carelessness, physical laziness and an unsteady body are some of the reasons for the lack of inner peace. Recitation and contemplation on the sound *Om* is offered as a sure way to remove these disturbances. Furthermore, Patanjali suggests cultivation of friendship, compassion, joyfulness, meditation, control of breathing and imbibing the example of accomplished masters as a means to obtain stillness of the mind. When an individual is able to cleanse his mind of these disturbances, he becomes totally tranquil. Patanjali asserts that one of the outcomes of this masterful concentration is that the student of Yoga develops the power of penetrating into the mysteries of both the inner and outer worlds. In *sutra* 40, it is clearly pointed out that the individual develops control over the smallest particle and the largest object in the universe. Though this extraordinary power of concentration may appear alien to us, part of it is exemplified by the lives of geniuses like Newton and Einstein. Through their extensive study and scholarship, both of these scientists developed a deep contemplative power to penetrate into the depths of the universe and were able to come up with equations that encapsulated the mystery of the cosmos in terms of its tiniest atom and the largest galaxy. If these human beings are fair examples of the dormant powers available to human beings, then the view of the Yoga philosophy about the existence of such powers is not out of place.

First stage of mental stillness

1.41 When mental fluctuations are brought under control, consciousness shines like a clear crystal, which by reflecting the true nature of the knower, the instrument of knowing and the known identifies itself with each.

Commentary This important *sutra* links the earlier ones dealing with mental fluctuations and the later ones describing stages of mental stillness. Our ordinary mind is like a stained mirror incapable of reflecting the true nature of the object put before it. Once the mirror is cleansed of these stains, it can reflect the object without distortions. Similarly, since the everyday worries, anxieties, concerns and fears muddy our mind, it is incapable of reflecting the true light of the inner self (*Purusha*). Once these tainting fluctuations are brought to a standstill and the mind is cleansed of their dirtying impediment, it becomes like a clear mirror, which can reflect anything that is put before it whether it is the object or the instrument of knowing or the knowing subject. Devoid of these mental fluctuations, the mind can now reflect the true nature of anything that is placed before it.

Furthermore, this cleansing of fluctuations brings the mind to the threshold of its own contents and workings. The *Sutras* that follow describe different levels of mental stillness achieved when concentration is focused on various aspects of the mind. Since each one of these levels of contemplative consciousness (*samadhi*) deals with a different content of the mind it is given a special name.

✱Higher levels of mental stillness or tranquillity (involution)

1.42 The stage of mental stillness called *savitarka samadhi* is achieved when consciousness attains knowledge of an object by blending together the word, meaning and content.

1.43 In the next stage of mental stillness, called *nirvitarka samadhi*, consciousness cleansed of memory and its own nature reveals the object in its true nature without any distortions from the intermingling of word or meaning.

1.44 Now the contemplative consciousness moves onto the higher reflective stage of stillness called *savicara samadhi*. Here the focus of contemplation is subtle objects only. In the next level of super-contemplation, called *nirvicara samadhi*, consciousness is even devoid of thought.

1.45 In the next stage, contemplative consciousness moves beyond all manifested subtle objects and meditates on their cause, the subtlest unmanifest objective reality (*Prakriti*).

1.46 The earlier four stages of contemplative consciousness are called mental stillness with seed (*sabija samadhi*).

1.47 By attaining the super-reflective stillness (*nirvicara samadhi*), there is the dawning of utmost spiritual clarity.

1.48 Here, consciousness becomes truth bearing wisdom.

1.49 This truth bearing wisdom is called intuitive knowledge because it is gained without the help of testimony or inference.
1.50 The impressions produced by the truth bearing wisdom destroy all old ones and stop new ones from arising.
1.51 When the impressions of truth bearing wisdom are also destroyed, then the seedless stage of mental stillness (*nirbija samadhi*) arises.

Commentary In the commentary on the *samprajnata* and *asamprajnata samadhis*, it was pointed out that once the student of Yoga is able to cut off connection with the external world through the tools of practice and non-attachment, she is ready to embark upon a journey into the inner world of consciousness. During this excursion, the student's contemplative consciousness moves through seven stages called *samadhis*. In the *samprajnata samadhi*, the student concentrates on reasoning, reflection, joy and ego-sense, whereas in the *asamprajnata samadhi*, the contemplative consciousness transcends these four mental activities. In *Sutra* 42, Patanjali reintroduces the subject of *samadhi* by going deeper into levels of consciousness, naming them *savitarka, nirvitarka, savicara, nirvicara* and *nirbija samadhis*. In *savitarka samadhi*, contemplative consciousness concentrates upon the knowledge of the object, but attains it at a higher level by blending together the word, meaning and content. Similarly, in *nirvitarka samadhi*, contemplative consciousness cleansed of all memory of its past contents, including language and its own nature, achieves knowledge of the object without the aid of word or meaning. As the stillness of the mind is enriched through these levels of concentration, the student undertakes the next difficult task of *savicara samadhi*. Here consciousness reflects on the nature of the ego-sense and how it causes the sense of individuation as well as the distortion of mixing one's real self with the ego-self. Once this is accomplished, contemplative consciousness moves beyond the sense of I-am-ness as well as the trappings of both language and thought to a super-contemplative state. After transcending all objects, their causes and thought, consciousness concentrates on *Prakriti*, the subtlest cause of everything that exists.

Patanjali calls these four levels of contemplative consciousness *sabija samadhi* because all of them are still focused on some kind of object whether material or subtle. Once this state of stillness of the mind is gained, the aspirant's consciousness becomes the truth bearing wisdom or intuitive knowledge because it transcends all the ordinary ways of knowing. At this stage, while shining in its own purest nature, intelligence (*buddhi*), which gains wisdom through the direct apprehension of reality, is still only the reflection of *Purusha*. In the next stage called *nirbija samadhi*, when all fluctuations including the experience of the truth bearing wisdom are transcended, *Purusha* shines forth as the pure witnessing consciousness. This is the state of total stillness of the mind called variously the state of complete bliss or peacefulness, or enlightenment.

CHAPTER NINE

Sadhanapada: the method of Yoga

This part, consisting of 55 *sutras,* deals with two distinctive and yet related aspects of the Yoga method. The first, called *Kriya Yoga,* is presented as a preliminary method for the initiate whose mind is distracted by various afflictions. Through the control and elimination of these obstacles, this method prepares the student for the stillness of the mind. The second method, which is called *Ashtanga Yoga,* consists of eight steps. It is meant for the serious student who wants nothing less than enlightenment. This method, when perfected, leads the individual to total freedom from all limitations or salvation.

Sutras

Kriya Yoga: the Yoga of action

2.1 Self-discipline, self-study and self-surrender constitute the preliminary Yoga or the Yoga of action (*Kriya Yoga*).
2.2 The practice of this Yoga reduces the effectiveness of afflictions (*kleshas*) and prepares the way for the stillness of the mind.

Commentary In the earlier part, Patanjali uses the phrase 'mental fluctuations' (*chitta-vrittis*) to designate all disturbances in the ordinary mind that hinder the full expression of *Purusha,* and he sets forth the goal of Yoga as the stilling of these fluctuations. It is quite obvious from the discussion in the previous chapter that since these mental fluctuations arise from different ways of knowing, they are epistemological in nature. However, in Part II, Patanjali introduces a second set of disturbances called afflictions (*kleshas*). Unlike fluctuations (*chitta-vrittis*), afflictions (*kleshas*) appear to be both epistemological and ethical in nature. In contrast to mental fluctuations they are imperfections embedded in one's personality, which need to be worked on diligently by the student of Yoga. Patanjali suggests a unique method of *Kriya Yoga* that aims to minimize their effectiveness by reducing them to their dormant state.

The method of *Kriya Yoga* consists of self-discipline (*tapas*), self-study (*svadhyaya*) and self-surrender (*Ishwara-pranidhana*). Its goal is to produce stillness of the mind through the purification of three aspects of the personality. It aspires to improve the person through the formation of good habits of the body, speech and mind. The first step of self-discipline (*tapas*) is directed towards the recovery of the body and mind from their dependence on the external world.

Through self-discipline, the student of Yoga decides to take a careful note of the appetites and desires through which she clings to the world. Once these dependencies are understood, the student attempts to burn away these impurities through the living of a simple and austere life. Patanjali suggests the use of prayer, self-control and understanding as effective means of lessening one's reliance on these habitual addictions.

Self-discipline is enhanced by the second step of self-study (*svadhyaya*). Here the student takes an inventory of every aspect of one's personality including one's needs, desires and wants. One adopts an objective view of these needs by scrutinizing the way one organizes one's life around them. Some of these needs are found to be genuine because our life depends upon them while others are superficial because we have acquired them without much scrutiny. As we become able to separate these two kinds of needs, we also stop identifying our real self with them. Patanjali suggests recitation of sacred words, imbibing the lives of accomplished Yogis and reading sacred books as aids to self-understanding.

The third step of self-surrender (*Ishwara-pranidhana*), which aims to minimize the stronghold of the ego on one's personality, enriches the other two steps. Through self-discipline and self-study, the student of Yoga realizes the power of the ego in creating our separateness from others. The ego's emphasis on individuality leads to acquiring things for oneself and safeguarding them from others. In self-surrender, one reverses this approach by lessening the hold of the ego through the cultivation of compassion for others as well as through developing a more intimate sense of connection with the universe. In order to facilitate this transition, one follows certain rules of behaviour. Giving rather than taking becomes one's motto. One acts and does everything not for oneself but for others or for the sake of a higher being who is regarded as the underlying connecting reality. Instead of asking things for oneself, one seeks them out for others. As one lets go of one's attachment to things, one stops identifying with the artifacts of the world. The adoption of these three steps helps the student come closer to achieving peacefulness of the mind.

The method of *Kriya Yoga* is intended for both the novice and the more serious student of Yoga.

Kleshas: five afflictions of body, emotions and mind

2.3 The afflictions (*kleshas*) are ignorance (*avidya*), egoism (*asmita*), attachment (*raga*), repulsion (*dvesha*) and clinging to life (*abhinivesha*).

2.4 Ignorance (*avidya*) is the breeding ground for the other four afflictions whether they are in their dormant, weakened, interrupted or fully operative states.

2.5 Ignorance lies in taking the non-eternal as eternal, the non-real as real, the painful as pleasurable and the non-self as self.

2.6 Egoism is the identification of the seer with the seen.

2.7 Attachment is intense craving after pleasure.

2.8 Repulsion is caused by the fear of pain.
2.9 Intense clinging is a natural affliction present even in the wise.
2.10 Through the practice of *Kriya Yoga*, the active afflictions can be transformed into dormant ones.
2.11 Both dormant and subtle afflictions can be subdued through meditation.

Commentary Here Patanjali introduces five afflictions (*kleshas*) that are deeply rooted in the human existence. Every person's body and mind are inflicted with imperfections of ignorance (*avidya*), egoism (*asmita*), attachment (*raga*), repulsion (*dvesha*) and clinging to life (*abhinivesha*).

The first two afflictions of ignorance and egoism are flaws of the mind. Through ignorance a person mistakes the real for the unreal, the self for the non-self and the pleasurable for the painful. This is exemplified through our attitude towards our true self. Most of us believe that we are nothing more than the body-mind complex and ignore the existence of pure consciousness or *Purusha*, which is our true essence. Part of this ignorance is also evident when we confuse our true, eternal self with the ego, which is part of the non-eternal and perishable psychophysical self.

Ignorance and egoism are responsible for mental suffering, whereas emotional pain is a result of attachment (*raga*) and repulsion (*dvesha*). Most of us identify ourselves with our emotions. Through them we desire the world of objects, and become attached to them. We want these objects for ourselves and once we obtain them, we safeguard them from the encroachment of others. When under the sway of emotions we can be consumed by strong attachment to our possessions or by hatred of losing them to others.

The last affliction of clinging to life or intense fear of death (*abhinivesha*) is a natural fear of losing our body. It may manifest itself through the desire to prolong life and, if possible, to make it immortal. This desire may become so morbid that the individual will safeguard his life at all costs, causing havoc to his personal, social and professional life.

These five afflictions are the main causes of physical, mental and spiritual suffering. However, their effectiveness can be reduced by the practice of *Kriya Yoga* as well as meditation.

Suffering and emancipation: Bhagavad Gita and Samkhya

2.12 Accumulated effects of actions (*karmas*) of past lives are rooted in afflictions and are responsible for experiences of present and future lives.
2.13 This storehouse of effects of past actions (*karmas*) determines the class of birth, lifespan and experiences in one's present life. *Sanskaras*
2.14 The virtuous or vicious actions of the past result in joy or sorrow in this life.
2.15 Apprehending the influence of mental modifications, qualities of nature and effects of past actions, the discriminating person who knows that even

pleasant experiences are adulterated with pain remains indifferent to material objects.

2.16 Future suffering can be avoided.
2.17 Future suffering, which is due to the identification of the seer with the seen, can be eliminated.
2.18 The material universe, which is of the nature of joy, activity and inertia, is conducive to enjoyment or emancipation.
2.19 The three qualities of nature have the characteristics of being particular or universal, differentiated or undifferentiated.
2.20 The seer, who is pure consciousness, still sees with the instrument of the mind.
2.21 The material universe exists for the sake of the seer.
2.22 The objects of nature, which cease to exist for the emancipated ones, remain in existence for the unemancipated ones.
2.23 Because of association with the seen, the seer comes to an understanding of one's own nature.
2.24 Ignorance is the cause of the false identification of the seer and the seen.
2.25 When the disassociation of the seer from the seen occurs, ignorance is destroyed and the seer is emancipated.
2.26 Continuous practice of discriminative knowledge leads to the destruction of ignorance.

Commentary   In these fifteen *Sutras* (2.12–2.26), Patanjali presents his position on reincarnation. His views about reincarnation are similar to the *karma* theory of the *Bhagavad Gita* and his views about suffering and the way to emancipation are similar to those of Samkhya. The *Bhagavad Gita* teaches that our present life is not an accident on this earth. It is rather due to the effects of actions (*karmas*) of our past lives. These results are rooted in afflictions, which are the main constructs of human existence on this earth. The consequences of actions of our past lives determine precisely our class of birth, lifespan and the pleasant and unpleasant experiences of our present and future lives. All the joys and sorrows of this life are determined by our deeds of the past.

When a student of Yoga grasps these influences and realizes that even the most pleasurable experience of this life is adulterated with pain, he learns to detach himself from craving objects of this world. This kind of understanding helps decrease both present and future suffering.

Furthermore, Patanjali accepts the Samkhya view, which holds ignorance as responsible for all suffering. Ignorance is due to mistaking the unreal for the real or the non-eternal for the eternal, or the non-self for the self. A person in ignorance falsely identifies the true self (*Purusha*) with the ordinary mind (*Prakriti*). Since *Purusha* sees the world with the agency of the ordinary mind, it is easy for the mind to undergo this kind of identification. Besides acting as a trap for *Purusha*, the mind is also the agent of its liberation. It is through the mind that *Purusha* witnesses the drama of the world of *Prakriti* and becomes aware of its own entrapment. Also it is through the mind that *Purusha* comes to know its own nature. When the student of Yoga realizes that he is *Purusha* and not *Prakriti,* this dawning of discriminative knowledge breaks the net of ignorance and the individual is emancipated. Patanjali suggests the eightfold path of *Ashtanga Yoga* to help the student develop discriminative knowledge and reach enlightenment.

The seven stages of discriminative knowledge

2.27 Discriminative knowledge develops through seven stages.

Commentary In *Sutra* 2.27, when Patanjali says that discriminative knowledge develops through seven stages, he might be suggesting two different things. First, he might be referring to the seven types of *samadhis* discussed earlier as seven stages of discriminative knowledge. Second, he might be referring to the first seven steps of *Ashtanga Yoga,* which are arranged as seven hierarchical stages of discriminative knowledge leading to the final step of complete stillness of the mind or *samadhi.*

Ashtanga Yoga: eight steps of the Yoga method

2.28 The practice of the different steps of the Yoga method leads to the removal of all impediments and results in discriminative knowledge or illumination.

2.29 Restraint (*yama*), discipline (*niyama*), physical posture (*asana*), regulation of vital force (*pranayama*), sense-organ withdrawal (*pratyahara*), concentration (*dharana*), meditation (*dhyana*) and absorption (*samadhi*) are the eight steps of Yoga.

Commentary Here Patanjali is introducing the method of *Ashtanga Yoga,* which is the experiential-scientific way of achieving discriminative knowledge or enlightenment. This method consists of eight steps arranged in a hierarchical order. The first five are aimed at controlling the influences of the external world, whereas the last three are focused on cleansing the contents of the ordinary mind.

The first step offers five restraints (*yamas*) of non-violence, non-lying, non-stealing, non-craving for sexual pleasure and non-possessiveness as moral principles to be mastered. The second step embraces five disciplines (*niyamas*) of purity, contentment, austerity, self-study and ego-surrender as positive principles of physical and mental hygiene. By building proper habits of the body and mind, the individual becomes fully focused to undertake the difficult task of the purification of her entire personality. These ten rules of physical and mental control prepare the student for the arduous inward journey.

Once these mental attitudes are cultivated, the student is ready to move on to the next two steps of physical posture (*asana*) and breath control (*pranayama*). These two aim to perfect every part of the body as well as to control all emotions. Physical postures cleanse the body of all impurities so that it becomes disease-free and, if possible, ageless. However, through the voluntary control of inhalation, retention and exhalation, breathing exercises regulate the intake of the life force. Their goal is to cleanse the lungs as well as the heart. Since our emotions are dependent upon our lungs, heart and breathing, through regulation we can develop mastery over them.

These four steps help the student develop control of influences arising from the external world of people and objects. However, the individual has yet to learn to discipline the five sense organs, which supply all information arising from the outer world. In the fifth step, *pratyahara*, the student cuts off all contact between the sense organs and their objects by withdrawing consciousness inward. This is the final step, which marks the development of total mastery over the influences of the outside world. Now the student of Yoga is ready to undertake the most difficult task of cleansing the contents of the mind through the three inner meditative steps, which are discussed in detail in Part III of the *Yoga Sutras*. Once the individual washes his mind of all mental impurities, he achieves total stillness, also called enlightenment.

Ten principles of physical and mental hygiene

2.30 The restraints (*yamas*) are non-violence, non-lying, non-stealing, non-craving for sexual pleasure and non-possessiveness.

2.31 Class, place, time and circumstance do not limit the five restraints.

2.32 The disciplines (*niyamas*) are purity, contentment, self-discipline, self-study and self-surrender.

2.33 When one's mind is shaken by disturbing thoughts, one should concentrate on opposites.

2.34 Actions of violence done by oneself or got done by others or approved by oneself originate in greed, anger or ignorance. Because they can be mild, medium or intense, and result in endless suffering, reflection on the opposites is necessary.

2.35 Habitual indulgence in non-violence leads to the termination of hostility in the presence of others.

2.36 When a person is established in truth, such a person's words bear their fruits.

2.37 When a person is firmly established in non-stealing, fortunes are showered on this person from all directions.

2.38 When one is firmly established in sexual control, one gains intense vigour.

2.39 When one frees oneself from possessions, one gains knowledge of past and future lives.

2.40 When the cleanliness of the body is cultivated, disinclination towards self-gratification through contact with others is developed.

2.41 When the body is cleansed, the mind is unsullied and the senses are disciplined, one achieves joyful wisdom of the inner self.
2.42 When contentment is cultivated, supreme happiness arises.
2.43 When self-discipline is perfected and impurities are destroyed, and perfection of sense organs and the body results.
2.44 When self-study is practised, one gains access to the inner self.
2.45 When one's ego is surrendered, one attains the state of mental stillness.

Commentary The five restraints (*yamas*) of non-violence, non-lying, non-stealing, non-craving for sexual pleasure and non-possessiveness and the five disciplines (*niyamas*) of purity, contentment, austerity, self-study and ego-surrender comprise the ten commandments for the student of Yoga. Patanjali gives prominence to non-violence by regarding it as the basic principle underlying the other four restraints. Since violence in any form is destructive, it is the root cause of all personal, social and spiritual suffering. In contrast, non-violence is based upon the principle of sanctity of life. Its habitual practice in thought, speech and action results in the termination of all hostility towards others. Moreover, non-violence leads to truthfulness, non-stealing, non-craving for sexual pleasure and non-possessiveness.

According to Patanjali, the adoption of these ten commandments result in many beneficial consequences for the individual. When the attitude of non-stealing is cultivated, wealth comes to such a person; when one develops control over sexual desire, one gains royal vigour; when one practises contentment, supreme happiness is the outcome; and when one seriously indulges in introspection, one gains knowledge of the inner self.

The sceptics among us might doubt the practicality of these Yoga commandments, but we do have Mahatma Gandhi and Martin Luther King as two outstanding examples of followers of the first two Yoga rules. Mahatma Gandhi perfected the rules of non-violence and truthfulness by transforming them into a political tool, with which he was able to persuade the British to end their colonial rule in India. Similarly, Martin Luther King adopted the principles of non-violent resistance to fight racism and inequality in the United States. His actions brought about beneficial consequences. Bishop Desmond Tutu, who advocated non-violence as a tool to end apartheid in South Africa, is another living example of the Yoga emphasis on non-injury and respect for life.

Physical postures and breathing exercises

2.46 Posture (*asana*) should be firm and easy.
2.47 Posture reaches perfection when it is performed effortlessly.
2.48 When posture is mastered, dualistic thinking comes to an end.
2.49 The regulation of inhalation, retention and exhalation of breathing or the life force (*pranayama*) is the next step.

2.50 The inhalation, exhalation and retention of breathing are precisely regulated according to place, time and number so that breathing becomes subtle and prolonged.
2.51 The fourth aspect of the control of life force goes beyond both inhalation and exhalation.
2.52 When the regulation of the life force is mastered, the veil of ignorance is weakened.
2.53 Then the mind calms down and is prepared for concentration.

Commentary The Yoga system believes that our body is the field for the growth of the spirit. If the field lacks the proper nutrients or is unhealthy, the full expression of the spirit will be blocked. To make the body a perfect vehicle, it must be mastered through physical exercises. The Yoga system gives us 64,000 physical postures to perfect each part of the body so that it can become disease free and ageless, as well as a faultless reflector of the light of the spirit.

God *Shiva*, who mastered these 64,000 postures, is the prime example of the ageless master Yogi. Patanjali suggests that an individual can also derive the same kinds of benefits by practising physical postures on a regular basis and for a long time.

Along with the practice of physical postures, Patanjali recommends the regulation of the three breathing processes of inhalation, retention and exhalation. By disciplining breathing, one can develop control over the life force (*prana*), which brings about many beneficial consequences. Since our breathing purifies the blood and affects emotions and thinking, by regulating it one develops control of the states of the body and mind. A student who has learned voluntary control of the three phases of breathing can generate within herself any emotional state at will.

Research is being conducted at the Himalayan Institute in Honesdale, Pennsylvania, where researchers are trying to find a link between breathing from the left or right nostril and its direct effect on the right or left side of the brain. If the research establishes a conclusive connection between breathing through a specific nostril and a certain part of the brain, its practical application to human development will add another piece of supporting evidence to the Yoga claims regarding breathing control.

Total disconnection of senses from objects

2.54 Sense object withdrawal (*pratyahara*) is the next step, where senses are withdrawn from the objects and directed inward.
2.55 This results in the total control of the senses.

Commentary Once the first four steps are mastered, the influence of the outer world is minimized. Before undertaking the difficult task of meditation, Patanjali introduces the step of *pratyahara*, which aims to disconnect the sense organs from the influence of their respective physical objects. In this step, the senses are withdrawn from the objects and directed inward. Patanjali believes that all consciousness belongs to *Purusha*. Our knowledge of the physical world results when this consciousness is directed towards the ordinary mind, which directs it towards the sense organs, which, in turn, direct it towards the objects. In the *pratyahara* step, the mind reverses this process by withdrawing consciousness from the sense organs and directing it inward. This cuts off the connection between the senses and their respective objects. Though this is a very difficult step to learn, it can be mastered under the supervision of a teacher of Yoga.

Once this disconnection of the sense organs from their objects is perfected the student will be fully prepared to undertake the next arduous journey, which requires the mastery of the three inner steps of concentration.

CHAPTER TEN

Vibhutipada: accomplishments of Yoga

Vibhutipada, which consists of 56 *sutras*, is the longest of the four parts of the *Yoga Sutras*. Here Patanjali begins with a description of concentration (*dharana*), meditation (*dhyana*) and absorption (*samadhi*) as the three steps of meditation. The major portion of the text discusses the powers that a meditator achieves through the perfection of the meditative practice. These attainments are described as extraordinary or supernormal powers that result from the mastery of the steps of concentration. When an accomplished meditator concentrates on different aspects of himself, others or the universe, he obtains extraordinary knowledge and control over them. These supernormal powers range from knowledge of the past and the future, other minds, the solar system, the starry heavens and the language of animals to the power of levitation, walking on water, hearing celestial music and the like. Though many of these powers can be developed by the practice of Yoga, Patanjali cautions the student from becoming too attached to them because they are obstacles to the achievement of the final goal of Yoga.

Sutras

The three internal steps of meditation

3.1 Concentration (*dharana*) is the spontaneous directing of consciousness towards an object.
3.2 Meditation (*dhyana*) is the uninterrupted flow of consciousness towards an object.
3.3 Absorption (*samadhi*) is the uninterrupted merging of consciousness into an object where self-awareness is completely erased.
3.4 When concentration, meditation and absorption work together as a single contemplative process, it is called one-pointed attention (*samyama*).
3.5 When one-pointed attention (*samyama*) is perfected, the light of wisdom dawns.
3.6 One-pointed attention (*samyama*) can be practised on various aspects of life.
3.7 The three steps constituting one-pointed attention (*samyama*) are internal in contrast to the previous five, which are external.
3.8 When compared to seedless contemplation (*nirbija samadhi*), even these three steps are external.

Commentary Patanjali opens this part with the discussion of the three steps of meditation called concentration (*dharana*), meditation (*dhyana*) and absorption (*samadhi*). They are different stages of concentration ranging from the lowest to the highest.

In concentration (*dharana*), the mind of the individual is cut off from disturbances arising from the external world and is ready to take inventory of its own contents. Here the student chooses an image or an idea of his own liking and attends to it. As the individual focuses the mind on a single item, other ideas make their presence felt. The student must bring back his mind to the original idea and keep it there as long as he can. Since other ideas are distractions, the mind needs to be brought back again and again to the chosen idea. As concentration improves with practice, there are fewer and fewer distractions. When an individual is able to keep his mind on a chosen idea for a long time, this spontaneous concentration is called meditation (*dhyana*). Here the student is able to concentrate on any idea without distraction. The only distraction still present is one's awareness of oneself as a subject. With more practice this self-consciousness disappears and the individual becomes totally engrossed in the object of contemplation. This stage is called absorption (*samadhi*).

When these three stages work together as a team, they are called one-pointed attention (*samyama*). An accomplished student of Yoga while directing one-pointed attention towards himself, other people or the universe can reveal their innermost secrets. This capacity to unravel such mysterious knowledge, which is unavailable to the ordinary mind, is called extraordinary or supernormal power. Patanjali gives many examples of supernormal powers developed through the use of one-pointed attention.

Three mental transformations

3.9   Restraint transformation (*nirodha parinama*) is a change in consciousness, which becomes successively imbued with the state of stillness that temporarily mediates between outgoing and incoming impressions.
3.10 When this consciousness transformation maintains a steady awareness of the gap between the outgoing and the incoming impressions, tranquillity overflows.
3.11 Contemplative transformation (*samadhi parinama*) is that change where awareness moves from all-pointed to one-pointed consciousness.
3.12 Absorption transformation (*ekagrata parinama*) is that change where consciousness moves from one-pointed to no-pointed concentration.

Commentary   Sutras 9 to 12 are the most intriguing ones in this part. They have been given various interpretations by commentators.

The three meditative steps of concentration, meditation and absorption bring the student of Yoga to the threshold of the mind where one faces three corresponding transformations of consciousness called the restraint transformation (*nirodha parinama*), contemplative transformation (*samadhi parinama*) and absorption transformation (*ekagrata parinama*). These transformations should not be confused with static states because they are dynamic conditions of consciousness. In the restraint transformation (*nirodha parinama*), consciousness tries to suppress its own content by narrowing down its field of attention from many to one item only. When consciousness focuses on one object and then on its absence, it becomes aware of the silence of absence. As consciousness rests on this silence, residing between the two occurrences of the object, it tries to enhance the duration of this peaceful surge. When one can maintain this stream of serenity for a long time, one reaches the stage of contemplative transformation (*samadhi parinama*). Here consciousness becomes a one-pointed flow of tranquillity. As the student practises concentration on the emptiness of her own mind, she moves from one-pointed to no-pointed attention. This flow of consciousness devoid of all content is called dynamic void or the stage of absorption transformation (*ekagrata parinama*). Through these three transformations, the student moves from multi-pointed to one-pointed and then on to no-pointed concentration.

Three transformations in the world of objects

3.13 The three transformations of consciousness in terms of property, character and condition also happen in objects and sense organs.
3.14 The underlying substance holds together properties in their latent, manifest and unmanifest forms.
3.15 The distinctive transformations are due to the differences residing in the underlying substratum.

Commentary In *Sutra* 13, Patanjali points out that an accomplished student develops mastery over the workings of the mind through the three transformations of consciousness. Similarly, the same three techniques can be applied to the sense and motor organs as well as objects. This application of the meditative tools can help the student master the physical world of *Prakriti* as well as develop many supernormal powers.

In the next two *sutras*, Patanjali describes the nature of *Prakriti* as the underlying substance which is constituted of three qualities of good (*sattva*), activity (*rajasa*) and inertia (*tamasa*). Since all objects in the universe are constructed from the same three ingredients, every transformation that takes place in the sense and motor organs or in the world of objects is also due to the differences residing in the nature of this substratum (*Prakriti*).

One-pointed attention and extraordinary powers

3.16 By directing one-pointed attention (*samyama*) towards the transformation of property, character and condition, one gains knowledge of the past and the future.

3.17 When one-pointed attention (*samyama*) is directed towards the sound, meaning and idea components of language, one gains the knowledge of sounds produced by all living creatures.

Commentary To grasp the significance of the *Vibhutipada*, it is vital that we understand the meaning of two central terms: *samyama* and *siddhis*. Samyama has been translated variously as yogic contemplation, total concentration, insight, foresight, one-pointedness and one-pointed attention. Though all these meanings have been implied here, we will use the phrase 'one-pointed attention', which is the power of utmost concentration possessed by an accomplished student of meditation. Because this concentration has a laser-like precision, when it is directed towards anything it unravels the mystery of that object.

The second term *siddhis* has also been translated variously as accomplishments, attainments, achievements, extraordinary powers and supernatural or supernormal abilities. We will use it to designate extraordinary powers that are not within the grasp of people operating at the level of the ordinary mind. When a student masters the eight steps of the Yoga method, he develops extraordinary understanding that surpasses the capabilities of the ordinary mind. Most people use less than 10 per cent of their mind's capacity because this much utilization of mental power is sufficient to function effectively in the world. When, by utilizing only slightly more than 10 per cent of the mind's capability, geniuses like Newton and Einstein are able to unravel some of the major mysteries of the universe, it stands to reason that much more could be accomplished if we used a bigger chunk of our own minds.

Since the aim of Yoga is nothing less than the development and deployment of the total power of the mind, the aspirant attempts to accomplish this goal through the mastery of both the external and internal steps of the Yoga method. As the student develops into an accomplished meditator, he is able to utilize more of his mental capacities and thus attains a deeper understanding of the workings of the universe. This all-encompassing knowledge leading to the development of certain powers is a natural outcome of the mental growth resulting from the perfection of the Yoga practice. However, to the ordinary mind these powers seem to be extraordinary or supernormal in nature. As Patanjali outlines some of these powers, he also cautions the accomplished student not to become distracted by them because they will hinder progress towards enlightenment.

In *Sutra* 16, Patanjali holds that when one-pointed attention is directed towards the transformations of property, character and condition of an object, one attains knowledge of the past and the future. Here emphasis is put on transformations which, when attended to, will unravel the mystery of time. When the three transformations are under the laser-like scrutiny of concentration, the nature of the three aspects of time is grasped.

In *Sutra* 17, Patanjali points out that when an accomplished student directs her concentration towards the sound, meaning and concept components of language, she comes to understand the meaning of sounds produced by all living creatures. Suppose a lion is looking for his mate and is producing a growling sound. The sound involves an image of a mate plus the desire for intimacy. These three make up the complexity of that sound produced by the lion. An accomplished student of Yoga directs her attention to this complexity and is able to understand the sound, its meaning and its concept. This knowledge of the sound helps the student to understand the meaning of sounds produced by all living creatures.

Extraordinary powers and mental contents

3.18 When one-pointed attention (*samyama*) is directed towards past impressions, one obtains knowledge of previous lives.
3.19 When one-pointed attention (*samyama*) is directed towards ideas in one's own mind, one attains knowledge of one's mind as well as the minds of others.
3.20 When one-pointed attention (*samyama*) is directed towards an impression in another's mind, one gets knowledge only of the present mental content and not of the reason behind it.

Commentary In the above *Sutras*, Patanjali is describing three kinds of powers available to the accomplished student of Yoga. If concentration is directed towards the past impressions in one's own mind, one will be able to grasp one's previous lives. This can be explained through the theory of reincarnation. We are what we have done in this and in our past lives. All the impressions of our past are stored in our minds. When an accomplished student of Yoga concentrates on that part of the mind, he will be able to remember all of his past lives. Furthermore, when one-pointed attention is directed towards ideas in one's own mind, the accomplished meditator will be able to obtain knowledge of one's own mind as well as those of others. Moreover, by concentrating on an impression in another person's mind one can obtain the knowledge of the other's mind.

Sceptics might doubt the presence of such abilities in the trained student of Yoga. However, there are some people in our society who claim to have developed the power of clairvoyance through which they can read others' minds. These people call themselves psychics because they are able to penetrate into another's mind to unravel hidden secrets. Moreover, there are some excellent counsellors and psychotherapists who, by listening to their patients' problems, can identify with their inner world of emotions and through empathy can experience the meaning of their worries and anxieties. If these examples from ordinary life indicate the possibility of the existence of such powers, then it is feasible that accomplished students of Yoga have the ability to gain them through their strict practice.

Different kinds of extraordinary powers

3.21 When an accomplished student directs one-pointed attention (*samyama*) towards the bodily form, and breaks the contact between the light coming from the body and the eye, he can make the body invisible.

3.22 In a similar manner, by directing one-pointed attention (*samyama*) towards sound or smell, one can make them disappear.

3.23 By directing one-pointed attention (*samyama*) to the accumulated effects of actions of past lives (*karma*), one gains foreknowledge of death.

3.24 When one-pointed attention (*samyama*) is directed to the qualities of friendliness and fellowship, one strengthens these attributes.

3.25 When one directs one-pointed attention (*samyama*) to the power of animals, one gains the strength of an elephant.

3.26 By directing one-pointed attention (*samyama*) to the subtle, hidden and remote, one gains knowledge of them.

3.27 When one-pointed attention (*samyama*) is directed towards the sun, one attains knowledge of the solar system.

3.28 When one-pointed attention (*samyama*) is directed towards the moon, one gains knowledge of the starry heavens.

3.29 When one-pointed attention (*samyama*) is directed towards the Pole Star, one attains knowledge of the movement of the stars.

3.30 When one-pointed attention (*samyama*) is directed towards the solar plexus, one acquires knowledge of the entire body.

3.31 When one-pointed attention (*samyama*) is directed towards the throat, one feels no hunger or thirst.

3.32 By directing one-pointed attention (*samyama*) to the tortoise nerve (*kurma nadi*) complex, one achieves perfect steadiness.

3.33 When one-pointed attention (*samyama*) is directed to the light residing at the crown of one's head, one has a vision of the perfected beings.

Commentary   In the above *Sutras*, Patanjali describes various powers that can be achieved when one-pointed attention is directed to light, sound, effects of past actions and qualities of friendship and fellowship. When an accomplished student of Yoga fixes attention on the bodily form, and breaks the connection between the eye and the light coming from the body, he can make the body disappear. Similarly, through concentration, he can make sound, smell and taste disappear. Furthermore, when one-pointed attention is focused on the effects of the actions of past lives, one can gain knowledge of the time of one's death.

One-pointed attention is a perfect mental tool to gain knowledge about any part of the universe. In *Sutras* 24 to 33, Patanjali describes the special knowledge and supernormal powers gained by an accomplished student of Yoga who directs one-pointed attention to the quality of friendship; to the powers of animals; to the sun, the moon and the Pole Star; as well as to such parts of the human body as the solar plexus, the throat, the tortoise nerve and the light residing between the two eyes.

Other special powers of the mind and the body

3.34 When one-pointed attention (*samyama*) is directed to intuitive awareness, one gains knowledge of everything.
3.35 When one-pointed attention (*samyama*) is directed to the heart centre, one gains knowledge of consciousness.
3.36 When one-pointed attention (*samyama*) is directed to the higher self, one is able to grasp its true nature by distinguishing it from the lower self.
3.37 When one-pointed attention (*samyama*) is directed to the nature of the higher self, one gains extraordinary powers of hearing, touching, seeing, tasting and smelling.
3.38 These accomplishments are actually obstacles to the achievement of stillness of the mind (*samadhi*).

Commentary Patanjali portrays special powers that a student of Yoga can acquire through fixing one's mind on the appropriate parts of the body and on the mental contents. When one directs one-pointed attention towards the faculty of intuitive awareness, one obtains knowledge of everything. Furthermore, since Yoga thinkers believe that the higher self (*Purusha*) resides in the heart, if one fixes one's attention on it, one will be able to obtain knowledge of the nature of pure consciousness. Once this knowledge is gained, the student will be able to distinguish between the higher and lower self. By focusing one's attention on the nature of the higher self, one can acquire extraordinary abilities of hearing, touching, seeing, tasting and smelling.

After presenting these extraordinary powers as attainments of the accomplished student of Yoga, Patanjali offers a warning that these accomplishments could become obstacles to the attainment of the final goal of enlightenment. Students who have not yet learned full control of anger, fear and egoism might misuse these powers for personal aggrandizement, which could be a setback to achieving enlightenment.

Extraordinary bodily powers

3.39 By destroying the connection with the accumulated effects of past actions and having insight into the laws of the mind, one is able to enter another person's body.
3.40 By directing one-pointed attention (*samyama*) to the vital breath (*udana*), one is able to levitate as well as walk over water, mud and thorns.
3.41 By directing one-pointed attention (*samyama*) to the current of vital force of fire (*samana*), one develops an aura of light around oneself.

3.42 When one-pointed attention (*samyama*) is directed to the distinction between space and the power of hearing, one hears cosmic or divine melodies.

3.43 When one-pointed attention (*samyama*) is directed towards the relationship between the body and space, one develops the power to fly through space.

Commentary   In this section, Patanjali outlines a number of supernormal powers. However, he mentions the power of levitation twice. For the student of Yoga the power to levitate is a natural outcome of certain breathing exercises. Since we have been brought up in the scientific age, levitation may appear to be beyond credence. But we do have some examples where this power can be brought to the realm of credibility. Scientists have created simulators where astronauts in training float around in space suits, thus defying the law of gravity. We are amazed but believe it because science can explain this particular phenomenon. Similarly, the sages of Yoga have also worked out the connection between breathing and gravity. They believe that breathing is part of the cosmic force through which everything is connected. In human beings, breathing or life force manifests itself in five ways, one of which is connected to gravity. A student who has mastered the art of breathing exercises (*pranayama*) develops the capacity to levitate. An accomplished aspirant learns to direct her one-pointed attention to the vital force (*udana*) part of her breathing process, which makes her weightless and enables her to defy the gravitational constraint and levitate.

For the sake of clarity, we can also draw interesting parallels with some of the characters from the *Star Wars* films. Training of the Jedi Knights and the powers of Yoda can be compared to the Yoga practice and powers gained through it. Jedi Knights such as Obi-Wan Kenobi and Luke Skywalker were given training to teach them to feel the presence of the Force within and around. Their training involved rigorous physical and psychological exercises (similar to the first five steps of the Yoga method); meditation for long periods of time (similar to the three meditative steps); and unlearning what they had previously learned through eyes and ears (similar to the elimination of all mental fluctuations). Just like the accomplished students of Yoga, when the Jedi Knights had successfully completed their training, they came to possess certain powers of levitation and the ability to move objects from a distance.

Yoda, who was also trained as a Jedi Knight, became a Jedi master. Like a Yoga sage, Yoda could defy the ageing process. When he first met Luke Skywalker, he was already 900 years of age. He is represented as having big ears and big eyes. They might signify the two perceptual tools through which he had unlearned the information of his upbringings as well as the instruments through which he had trained himself to be in touch with the Force. The experience of the Force through rigorous training helps the Jedi Knight to develop many powers. Yoda constantly warns his Jedi students to beware of the lure of the dark side of the Force. 'A Jedi uses the Force for knowledge and defense, never for attack', is one of Yoda's maxims. Similarly, Yoga masters are constantly cautioning their disciples not to be lured by the extraordinary powers because they will hinder progress towards the realization of the ultimate force – the real self (*Purusha*).

Other supernormal powers

3.44 When one-pointed attention (*samyama*) is directed towards the disembodied state of consciousness, one destroys the veil that hides illumination.
3.45 When one-pointed attention (*samyama*) is directed towards mass, form, subtlety, conjunction and purpose of the elements, one gains mastery over them.
3.46 Through the control of these elements, one acquires powers of becoming minute, light, heavy, etc.
3.47 Graceful form, beauty, strength and diamond-hard constitution are the ingredients of a perfect body.

Commentary Our ordinary mind is infested with fluctuations arising from both the bodily and the psychological functions. They hide the light of pure consciousness or the true self. When a student of Yoga concentrates on the ordinary mind and divests it of distractions, he experiences the illumination of the true self.

In the next *Sutra*, Patanjali describes the way to gain knowledge as well as mastery over the elements of the universe. Everything is constructed from the elements of earth, water, fire, air and ether. They have the characteristics of mass, form, subtlety, conjunction and purpose. When an accomplished student of Yoga fixes her attention on these five characteristics, she understands the nature of these elements, and through this knowledge gains mastery over them. Furthermore, since one's body is made up of these five basic elements, through concentration, one acquires knowledge and control over them. This extraordinary knowledge prompts the ability in the student to transform his body into any shape from the smallest particle to the largest body. Once one gains total control of one's body, one can give it graceful form, beauty, strength and diamond-hard constitution which are the ingredients of a perfect body.

More unusual powers and enlightenment

3.48 When one-pointed attention (*samyama*) is directed towards the activity of perceiving, the ego-sense and the functions of sense organs, one gains mastery over them.
3.49 At this stage, without the use of sense organs, the mind is able to gain instantaneous cognition and mastery over the material reality.
3.50 One who knows the difference between the intelligence (*buddhi*) and the pure consciousness (*Purusha*) attains power over all the states of existence as well as knowledge of everything.
3.51 Total freedom dawns upon one who has destroyed the seeds of bondage and has detached from these supernatural powers.

3.52 By detaching oneself from attraction or pride or temptations from higher powers in charge of celestial domains, one avoids the possibility of being soiled by evil again.
3.53 When one-pointed attention (*samyama*) is directed towards the present moment and the succession of moments, one gains the highest knowledge, which is independent of the limitations of space and time.
3.54 Through this highest knowledge one gains the discriminative ability to distinguish between similars, which are indistinguishable in terms of class, character or position.
3.55 The highest knowledge, which is transcendent in nature, cognizes all objects at once and processes of the past, present and future concurrently.
3.56 Total enlightenment is achieved when the clarity of the intelligence (*buddhi*) equals that of the pure consciousness (*Purusha*).

Commentary These last nine *Sutra*s describe the highest powers acquired by the student of Yoga. The aspirant becomes so accomplished that by directing her one-pointed attention towards sense organs and the ego-sense, she gains mastery over them. Furthermore, she does not need to use the sense organs because her mind has become so powerful that it can cognize anything instantaneously. In this stage, an aspirant who knows the difference between intelligence (*buddhi*) and pure consciousness (*Purusha*) has all-encompassing knowledge and control over everything. Patanjali gives a warning that total freedom will be bestowed upon only those who have detached themselves from the lure of these supernormal powers. By detaching oneself from attraction, pride and temptation, one can transcend the trappings of the pleasures of the moment, and reach beyond the limitations imposed by time and space. By leaving behind all the fluctuations and enticements, one's intelligence becomes so clear that its clarity matches that of the pure consciousness. Here the aspirant reaches the goal of her life by becoming one with the ultimate force or pure consciousness. This is the stage of enlightenment sought by many but achieved by few.

CHAPTER ELEVEN

Kaivalyapada: total liberation or salvation as the final goal

Kaivalyapada, which consists of 34 *Sutras*, is the shortest of the four parts. Though it is slightly more than half the size of the other parts, it has presented interpreters with their biggest challenge. Patanjali is very specific about the content of each of the first three parts. His descriptions of the five mental fluctuations, the five psychological afflictions, the two methods of Yoga and the powers resulting from the practice are clearly presented. However, in this last part, Patanjali assumes that the reader already knows some of the basic concepts of Yoga and, therefore, need not be spoon-fed again. Though the major focus of *Kaivalyapada* is the nature of enlightenment and the ways to achieve it, Patanjali starts this part with a discussion of four additional ways other than one-pointed attention that are responsible for attaining supernormal powers.

Sutras

Powers achieved through other sources

4.1 These powers can be achieved through birth, drugs, repetition of sacred words, austerity or contemplation.

Commentary Patanjali lists five different ways through which these supernormal powers can be acquired. In some people, these powers are innate because their deeds of previous lives endow them with physical and mental capabilities to display them spontaneously. Since they are predisposed to these potentialities, these individuals can express them effortlessly. Buddha, Jesus, Prophet Mohammed, Sai Baba and Ramakrishna, as well as a number of sages and prophets of the past, are examples of people who were born with these powers.

Another way one can acquire them is through the use of certain potent herbs or drugs. In India, there are ascetics who prefer to use herbs like ganja or hashish to alter their ordinary mind in order to glimpse the extraordinary consciousness. Though the use of these herbs offers a higher kind of experience, it is still regarded as inferior to that acquired through mantras, austerity or one-pointed attention (*samyama*). A number of artists and poets of the past, including Aldous Huxley, Baba Ram Dass and Jean-Paul Sartre of the twentieth century, have used drugs to alter their ordinary consciousness to enhance their creative talents.

The chanting of mantras is suggested as another way of reaching the threshold of higher consciousness. As sound-symbols, mantras can be used as tools to guide the student towards deeper layers of consciousness. Since mantras provide the user with total control over oneself, they are judged to be offering a superior kind of experience. Because the chanting of mantras is a sure way to reach higher realms of consciousness, both the Transcendental Meditation and the Hare Krishna movements have capitalized on this aspect of the method to sell their spiritual products.

Moreover, Patanjali assigns a special place to austerity (*tapas*) in the attainment of supernormal powers. Since austerity requires a thorough understanding of one's dependencies as well as a rigorous mental training to eliminate one's imperfections, it is preferred over the use of drugs. Austerity is one of the major methods used by monks belonging to the Zen, Tibetan Buddhist and Christian religions.

Though Patanjali describes these four ways of gaining supernormal powers, he prefers contemplative consciousness or one-pointed attention (*samyama*). He regards it as the best method because it helps the student to develop self-control as well as giving assurance of achieving enlightenment. Swami Rama, Maharishi Mahesh Yogi and a number of sages of India are excellent examples of this method.

Predisposition and powers

4.2   The deluge of natural predispositions causes the change from one plane of existence to another.
4.3   Incidental cause does not push natural tendencies into action; it only removes impediments from their natural expression.

Commentary   Here Patanjali is referring to the theory of reincarnation, which holds that our present existence is not the result of mere accident or circumstance, but of our deeds in past lives. Every aspect of our current life, including physical and psychological constitution or birth in a certain family or caste, is the outcome of effects of actions performed during innumerable lives lived in the past. We are born with predispositions that cannot be changed but can be channelled in accordance with their natural flow. Patanjali offers the example of a farmer who while irrigating different parts of the field does not stop the flow of water, but opens up a segment of the barrier to distribute water to another area. Similarly, an individual cannot modify these natural endowments but can direct them like the farmer.

The mind of the master meditator

4.4   A master meditator can experience the world in many ways by creating different kinds of perspectives (personalities) due to the presence of the ego.
4.5   The mind of the master meditator controls all the created perspectives (personalities).

4.6 The mind of the master meditator, which is born of contemplation, is free from all bondage.

Commentary The ego plays a crucial part in creating identity for the individual. As an outstanding actor, it can create many unique roles for itself. An individual can live at innumerable levels by creating many different personalities for oneself. For example, a person's ego can assist one to adopt the perspective of a child, an adult, a middle-aged man or woman, a brother, a sister, a father, a mother, a friend, a lover, a teacher and the like. An ordinary individual might find it difficult to enact these roles, whereas a master meditator can display all of them but at the same time can stay free of them.

Impressions of the past actions

4.7 The impressions of the past actions (*karmas*) of the sage are neither white nor black, whereas those of others are coloured.
4.8 The impressions of three kinds of action come to fruition when circumstances are favourable.
4.9 Because of the causal connection between impressions of past actions and memory, the effects of the past determine the present life despite the differences of birth, space and time.
4.10 The memories and impressions of the past have existed from the beginning because the desire to live is eternal.
4.11 Since desire and impressions are held together by cause and effect, as the former ceases the latter disappears too.
4.12 Both the past and the future exist in their latent form in the present moment.

Commentary The effects of the actions of the past are described through the use of white and black colours, where black refers to evil and white designates good. Since the actions of an ordinary person are imbued with desire and attachment, the effects of these are either good or bad, or in between the two. In contrast, since a sage acts without desire and attachment, the effects of her actions transcend these categories. Moreover, Patanjali believes that since the principle of causality is all pervasive, there is an intimate connection between our memory and effects of the past. We carry these impressions from one birth to another as our possessions. These impressions have always existed because the desire to live has been there eternally. Since desires and impressions of the past are related as cause to effect, if the former is eliminated, the latter also ceases to exist. Moreover, our present life is a drama of the forces of the past and those of the future. The past is present in the form of predispositions and potentialities, whereas the future is present in the form of desires and goals, which are yet to be realized. Therefore, both the past and future exist in their latent form in the eternal present.

Qualities of material reality and the mind

4.13 All manifest or unmanifest forms are constituted of the three qualities (*gunas*) of material reality.
4.14 Each object is unique because it is constructed from a special combination of the three qualities of material reality.
4.15 Objects remain unchanged even though different people view them differently.
4.16 Objects are not dependent on any mind. What will happen to them when they are not cognized by any mind?
4.17 Objects are known according to the biases of the mind perceiving them.

Commentary Everything in the universe is constructed from the three qualities of good (*sattva*), activity (*rajasa*) and inertia (*tamasa*). Since these three ingredients are in different proportions in various objects, each item in the universe is a unique combination of them. Though various minds take different perspectives, the objects remain independent of the perceiving mind. Each object is comprehended differently by the special presuppositions of the perceiver. Whatever expectations one brings into the perceiving act, that is the way the object is viewed.

Pure consciousness versus ordinary mind

4.18 The pure consciousness or the higher self (*Purusha*), being omniscient, always knows the mental fluctuations.
4.19 Because the mind is material and perceptible, it is not self-luminous.
4.20 The ordinary mind is not the seer and the seen at the same time.
4.21 If we assume the illumination of one mind by another, then we have to assume the illumination of the first by another and so on which will result in confusion.
4.22 Pure consciousness or the higher self when reflected through the medium of the ordinary mind becomes identified with the latter's modifications.
4.23 The ordinary mind, which is coloured by the perceived object and by the borrowed consciousness of the higher self, appears to be all knowing.
4.24 Ordinary mind, which is a network of innumerable desires, exists as a tool for the use of the higher consciousness.
4.25 Ordinary mind, which is capable of taking the form of the knower and the known, appears to be all knowing.

Commentary The above *Sutras* can be understood in the context of the Samkhya view of the universe. The Samkhya philosophers believe that *Purusha* and *Prakriti* are the two ultimate realities from which everything in the universe is constructed. All consciousness belongs to the real self (*Purusha*), whereas material reality (*Prakriti*) and all its psychophysical products are unconscious. A human being is a unique combination of both the pure consciousness (*Purusha*) and material reality (*Prakriti*).

The Samkhya philosophers compare the pure consciousness of the higher self (*Purusha*) to the light of the sun. When the sun's light is reflected through the moon, the latter starts to glow; when the moon's light is reflected through the water, the entire pond radiates; and when this same light falls on a wall, it is illumined. When a child looks at the wall, he might believe that the light is coming from the wall, but an adult will tell him that it is originating from the moon and a scientist will point out that even the light of the moon is also borrowed from the sun.

By utilizing the above metaphor, Samkhya points out that though the ordinary mind and the body are unconscious and operate on borrowed consciousness of the real self, they begin to believe that consciousness is their own property. The ordinary mind is made up of three psychological functions of intelligence (*buddhi*), ego-sense (*ahamkara*) and understanding (*manas*). Since intelligence (*buddhi*), as the finest product of the material reality (*Prakriti*), lies in close proximity, it reflects clearly and distinctly the consciousness of the *Purusha*. Ego-sense (*ahamkara*) as the active product of *Prakriti*, reflects *Purusha*'s consciousness as well as deludes the individual into believing that consciousness is its own property. Furthermore, it confuses the individual by asserting that it is the true self. On the other hand, understanding (*manas*), as the conceptualizing activity of *Prakriti*, activates both the sense and motor organs by supplying to them consciousness through which they reveal the external world. Moreover, understanding categorizes all the information obtained by the senses in their contact with the outer world. Though these three aspects of the ordinary mind (*chitta*) have only borrowed consciousness, they delude themselves by believing that consciousness is their property.

Since we are conditioned by our cultural upbringing to believe that our true self is nothing more than our psychophysical self, we ignore the existence of *Purusha* at the core of our being. This ignorance of our real nature and the false identification with the psychophysical self or the ordinary mind is the reason for all discontentment and suffering. The goal of Yoga is to destroy this false identification through discriminative knowledge which consists of grasping that one's true nature is pure consciousness (*Purusha*) and not the material components. Through this discriminative knowledge one realizes first that the pure consciousness (*Purusha*), which is omniscient and self-luminous when reflected through mental modifications, can identify itself with them. Second, the ordinary mind, which is responsible for this false identification, can be used as a tool by the pure consciousness to eliminate all mental fluctuations so that one's true self as pure consciousness can be experienced.

Discriminative knowledge and enlightenment

4.26 The achievement of this discriminative knowledge leads the ordinary mind towards the highest illumination.

4.27 While discriminative knowledge is taking its hold, the ordinary mind can still be distracted by some impressions of the past.

4.28 These distractions should be removed like other afflictions.

4.29 One who maintains a complete non-attached attitude towards this discriminative knowledge achieves the highest enlightenment, called the 'trance that showers virtue and merit' (*dharma mega samadhi*).

4.30 This results in freedom from all afflictions and impressions of past acts.

4.31 When all mental modifications are eliminated and infinite wisdom is achieved, the knowledge of the ordinary mind appears to be trivial.

4.32 When the 'trance that showers virtue' is realized, the mission of the three qualities of nature is completed.

4.33 As the three qualities of nature cease to function, changes in time in terms of past, present and future also cease to exist.

4.34 In the final stage of enlightenment (*kaivalya*), the three qualities of nature, having accomplished their goals, merge back into the material reality and the higher self shines in its true nature.

Commentary In the above *sutras*, Patanjali describes the connection between discriminative knowledge and enlightenment. Discriminative knowledge leads one to stop confusing the lower with the higher self. Because the accomplished student of Yoga has freed oneself of all mental fluctuations, one finds the knowledge conveyed by the ordinary mind to be trivial. Furthermore, having reached total stillness, the mind ceases to be influenced by the three qualities of material reality. This state of mind is called the 'trance that showers virtue'. Here the three qualities, having accomplished their goal, merge back into material reality (*Prakriti*), and pure consciousness (*Purusha*) shines in its own blissful glow.

Part III
Yoga and health

CHAPTER TWELVE

Yoga and healing: the medical connection

In the West, healing is associated with medical science and its link to any spiritual tradition is often completely ignored. Since science stays within the domain of what is observable and verifiable, it limits itself to regarding a human being as a combination of the body, senses and mind. Because of this limited view, science focuses on healing only the observable aspects of a human being and ignores the spiritual dimension. However, in the past, healing and spirituality were intimately connected. As history indicates, the greatest healers of humankind were people like Jesus and Buddha and, more recently, Gandhi and Mother Teresa. In India, all systems of philosophy, especially Yoga, were developed to heal the imperfections of human existence. Each offered its unique method as an antidote to alleviate suffering. Since medical science regards a human being as a combination of body and mind, it presents ways of healing only these components of a person. Yoga goes a step further. It views the entire person as constituted of the body and mind and also pure consciousness. The body and mind make up the psychophysical vehicle through which pure consciousness as the true self of a person expresses itself. Yoga does not contradict medical science, but adds to it a spiritual component. By regarding a human being as a unique combination of pure consciousness and psychophysical self, Yoga's goal of healing thus becomes the integration of the entire person. To achieve this total health, Yoga emphasizes the cleansing of the body of all diseases and of the mind of all mental disturbances. Once that is accomplished the body and mind are then converted into a perfect vehicle for the uninterrupted expression of pure consciousness of the true self.

Yoga suggests an eightfold method whose aim is the integrative healing of the person. It works on the perfection of physical, psychological, moral and spiritual aspects. The first five steps of the Yoga method focus on cementing the body, senses and mind so that they function as a unit. Both bodily health and mental well-being require that these parts be disease-free and function at their optimum levels. Yoga believes in the indissoluble connection of the body and mind to a common spiritual source. A modification in the mind can bring a corresponding change in our body. A mental state of fear, anger or happiness can generate a parallel change in a specific organ of the body. For example, when we are angry our breathing and heart are accelerated, and our body might quiver or shake. When we are entertaining a romantic encounter, our immune system might get a boost. Because of this intimate connection between the state of the mind and the condition of the body, Yoga asserts that whatever one thinks, so does one become. Since health and healing are closely connected to the state of one's mind, the first two steps of the method are aimed at cleansing the mind of its impurities by offering certain restraints as well as principles of physical and mental hygiene. The mastery of the five moral restraints of non-violence, non-lying, non-stealing, non-craving for sensual pleasure and non-possessiveness, and the five moral principles of purity, contentment, austerity, introspection and ego-surrender are offered as preparatory steps for the total healing of the body.

Once these preliminary moral attitudes are mastered, both the body and mind are prepared to undertake the challenge of the next step. Yoga suggests many physical postures that cater to the health of the body. These exercises provide the entire body with nourishment so that each part becomes disease-free and functions at its optimum level. The mastery of these postures restores natural vitality to each organ of the body, which is conducive to defying the disintegrative process of ageing.

The physical postures are aided by the next step – the control of the vital force or breathing. According to Yoga, our breathing is the pulsation of the life force in us. It is our direct link to cosmic energy. Furthermore, it is through breathing that our lungs pick up the cosmic energy and inject it into the blood, which in turn, through the agency of the heart, distributes it to both the body and the mind. Breathing affects the integration of the person in a number of ways. First, it picks up the cosmic force from the air and supplies it to the lungs so that the blood is purified. This enriched blood acts as the pulsating life force within a person. Second, breathing injects the life force to the heart which, through the enriched blood, takes the energy and distributes it proportionately to all organs of the body. Moreover, since the heart is the seat of emotions, by nourishing it, breathing also nurtures the emotional world. Third, breathing utilizes the right and left nostrils to tap into the life force. When breathing is done from a particular nostril it has a direct link to the right or left side of the brain. The vital energy so breathed is conveyed immediately to a particular part of the brain thus establishing an immediate link between the brain and the cosmic force. Fourth, it is through breathing that we form a direct connection to the cosmic vital energy and to the universe.

According to Yoga, these four integrative functions of breathing can be brought under voluntary control by mastering the three processes of inhalation, retention and exhalation. By controlling the inflow and outflow of the life force as well as developing control of the retention of air, one can learn to master one's emotions. An accomplished student of Yoga, who has perfected the retention aspect of breathing, can also reduce the activity of her heart and reduce oxygen consumption, thus slowing down the ageing process. Yoga also emphasizes the connection between breathing and gravitational pull. By mastering the *udana* aspect of breathing, an accomplished student of Yoga can defy gravity by transforming herself into a bundle of energy particles and through this skill can perfect the art of levitation.

The perfecting of the ten principles of moral restraints and mental hygiene, as well as the mastery of physical postures and breathing, offer the individual physical health, emotional control and mental readiness to undertake the task of restoration of the mind. The mind is an agitated cauldron of desires, wants, anxieties, worries, satisfactions, dissatisfactions, pleasures, pains, images, ideas, ignorance and knowledge with which we identify ourselves. They are the driving forces and we appear to be helpless before them. In the Yoga terminology, they are called fluctuations in the mind. Since we identify our real self with some or all of them at different times, this leads to pain and suffering. Yoga aims to stabilize the mind by first controlling these disturbances and then removing them one by one. Three steps of meditation are used to discipline, control and finally eliminate these disturbances.

Through meditation one learns about the nature of sensations, perceptions, images, thoughts, emotions and activities of the ego-sense, and their hold on a person's mind. Furthermore, it is also through meditation that one frees oneself from their enslaving influence. The more an individual is able to understand and eradicate these fluctuations, the more one is able to heal one's mind. Once all these fluctuations are brought to a standstill, the mind, which is cleansed of them, now reflects its pure nature and is thus healed.

In the system of Yoga, the perfection of the body and mastery of the mind are not goals in themselves, but only means to a higher goal of the realization of the true self. Healing is the perfection of the body, senses and the mind, and the freeing of the spirit from its false identification with the products of material reality. Healing thus involves mastery of the psychophysical self as well as the gaining of wisdom about one's true nature as pure consciousness. Total healing, which is the goal of Yoga, thus becomes the restoration of the entire person where the body is cleansed of all diseases, the mind is purified of all mental fluctuations, and the true self shines in its own light as a witness to the world. This state of the person involves total freedom from all limitations. Here, the healed person has become whole and holy.

CHAPTER THIRTEEN

Practical aspects of Yoga

In the past, scholars who have translated and commented on the *Yoga Sutras* of Patanjali have either completely ignored or given scanty importance to the practical aspects of yoga. This benign neglect has served the purposes of the popularizers of the Yoga method who, in their turn, have described the physical (*asanas*), breathing (*pranayama*) and meditation (*dhyana*) exercises without reference to their philosophical and religious foundations. In their zest for mass appeal and consumption these zealots of the practical aspects of Yoga have cut these exercises completely off from their philosophical and religious roots. However, in the *Yoga Sutras*, Patanjali devotes a major portion of *Sadhanapada*, the second part of the book, to the description of the practical method called *Ashtanga Yoga*. Through the discussion of this method, Patanjali reveals the significance of the physical, breathing and meditation exercises in perfecting the body as well as achieving stillness of the mind. Their regular practice paves the way for the gaining of clarity of the mind which is a necessary step towards enlightenment. Thus, in *Sadhanapada*, this intimate connection between theory and practice is clearly revealed. In my own teaching, research and practice, I have always regarded Yoga to be an integrative discipline where philosophy and practice are indissolubly connected.

Since *An Introduction to Yoga Philosophy* is written to meet the needs of an academic and student readership, it is not within the scope of the present text to elucidate all the major exercises. However, it is of utmost importance to describe a small group of basic physical postures and breathing and meditation exercises in order to introduce the beginning student to the significant role played by them in achieving enlightenment.

In this chapter I will illustrate some of the physical (*asanas*), breathing (*pranayama*) and meditation (*dhyana*) exercises through which the Yoga method attempts to perfect the body and mind of a person. In the first part on physical postures (*asanas*), I will describe eight positions which are chosen for their simplicity and ease of execution. They can be practised by anyone irrespective of age or previous exposure to Yoga. The exercises pertain to different parts of the body ranging from the toes to the head. Since toes are the most neglected part of the body, healing begins by paying attention to them first. Beginning with the toes, these exercises focus on feet, heels, legs, thighs, abdomen, chest, back, arms, neck, face and head. By working on major muscles, organs and bones, the postures provide a gentle massage to the entire body by nurturing it back to its natural state of flexibility and restfulness.

Each posture should be practised slowly and without any strain. At first, it is sufficient to spend close to a minute on each exercise. Once you get accustomed to the routine and develop preferences for certain exercises, spend more time on them. For the complete relaxation of the body all the postures are recommended. Just like eating, drinking and sleeping, they provide the necessary nourishment to the entire body. For maximum benefit, these postures should be done on an empty stomach and on a regular basis. Furthermore, the wearing of loose clothes and the use of a comfortable mat are helpful in the practice of these exercises.

One should set up a routine by choosing a particular time and a specific place to do these exercises punctually. Moreover, a good mental attitude is essential. Before starting the exercises, one should tell oneself that one is going to spend this time exclusively on oneself without distractions from telephone, TV, radio or visitors. Furthermore, a detached attitude is also vital to this very personal enterprise. One should empty one's mind of all expectations of positive or negative outcomes resulting from the practice of these positions. To derive maximum benefit, it is recommended that the practice should be continued uninterruptedly for a long time.

Physical exercises (*asanas*)

Starting position (Figure 1)

Step 1: Extend both of your legs in front of you and sit straight up. Your hips, back, neck and head should be erect.

Step 2: Rest your hands on the knees. Look straight in front of you. Close your eyes.

Step 3: As you inhale and exhale, observe the flow of your breathing. It should feel very good.

To prepare yourself for the first posture, stay in this position for a minute while you breathe in and out. Keep observing the flow of your breathing. It should feel very good. This is your starting position. You will return to it before you begin and after you end most of these exercises.

Posture 1

Kneeling posture: part I (Figures 2, 3 and 4)

Step 1: Kneel on the ground, and sit back on your feet. Let your hips rest on the heels. Keep your hips, back and head straight up. Rest your hands on your knees. Look straight in front. Close your eyes. While you inhale and exhale, observe the flow of your breathing. It should feel very good.

Step 2: Take your hands behind you and rest them flat on the ground. Let your head hang. Remember to breathe in and out while observing the flow of your breathing.

Step 3: Put your hands and elbows flat on the ground in front of your knees. Place your forehead in between your hands. Let your chest rest on your thighs. While you inhale and exhale, observe the flow of your breathing. It should feel very good.

Kneeling posture: part II

Step 1: This position is just like the previous one except that you sit with your heels up while your hips are resting on them. Keep your hips, back and head straight up. Rest your hands on your knees. Look straight in front. Close your eyes. While you breathe in and out, observe the flow of your breathing. It should feel good.

Step 2: Take your hands behind you and rest them flat on the ground. Let your head hang. Remember to breathe in and out while observing the flow of your breathing.

Step 3: Put your hands and elbows flat on the ground in front of your knees. Place your forehead in between your hands. Let your chest rest on your thighs. While you breathe in and out, observe the flow of your breathing. It should feel very good.

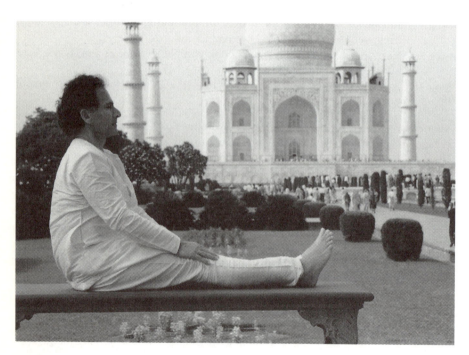

1   Starting position

Posture 2

Legs, arms and back stretch posture (Figure 5) Go back to the starting position as shown above. Keep your back, neck and head straight up. Let your hands rest on your knees. Breathe in and out while observing the flow of your breathing.

Step 1: Bring both your feet together. Move both feet closer to your body. They should be just far enough to be held comfortably by your hands.
Step 2: Surround your toes with both hands.
Step 3: Bend the upper part of your body so that your face touches your feet. Go down as far as you can. Do not strain yourself! Stay there for 30 seconds. Straighten out your back by sitting up. Extend your legs in front. Let your hands rest on your knees. Sit in the starting position.

Posture 3

Arms and back stretch posture: part I (Figure 6)

Step 1: While sitting in the starting position, move the left leg away from the right. Bend your right leg and move your right foot so that it rests against the left thigh.

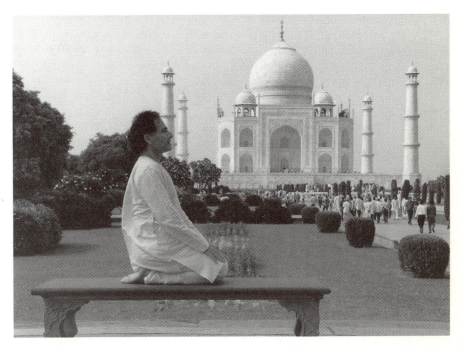

2 Kneeling position: step 1

Step 2: Hold on to the toes of the left foot with the left hand.
Step 3: Put your right hand over the left hand. Bend your body so that your face touches the left knee. Stay there for 30 seconds.

Arms and back stretch posture: part II (Figure 7)

Step 1: While sitting in the starting position, move the right leg away from the left. Bend your left leg and move your left foot so that it rests against the right thigh.
Step 2: Hold on to the toes of the right foot with the right hand.
Step 3: Put your left hand over the right hand. Bend your body so that your face touches the right knee. Stay there for 30 seconds.

Arms and back stretch posture: part III (Figure 8)

Step 1: While sitting in the starting position, keep both legs straight in front of you.
Step 2: Hold on to the toes with both hands.
Step 3: Bend your body so that your face touches your knees. Stay there for 30 seconds.

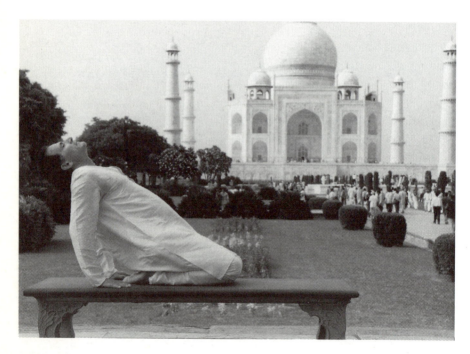

3 Kneeling position: step 2

Posture 4

Student's posture: part I (Figure 9)

Step 1: From the starting position, bend your right leg so that your right foot rests under your left thigh.
Step 2: Bend your left leg and gently move the left foot so that it passes over the right knee to rest on the ground. Now you are sitting on the right hip.
Step 3: Hold on to your left knee with the left hand and cover it with the right hand. Keep your back, neck and head straight up. While inhaling and exhaling, observe the flow of your breathing. It should feel very good.

Student's posture: part II

Step 1: From the starting position, bend your left leg so that your left foot rests under your right thigh.
Step 2: Bend your right leg and gently move the right foot so that it passes over the left knee to rest on the ground. Now you are sitting on the left hip.
Step 3: Hold on to your right knee with the right hand and cover it with the left

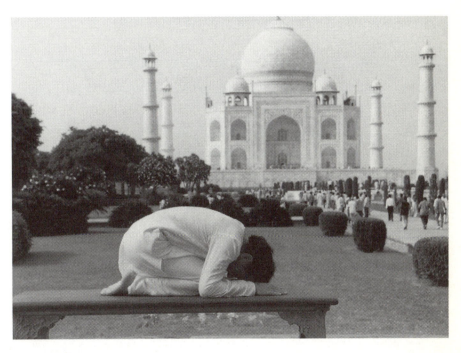

4 Kneeling position: step 3

Posture 5

Leg and back stretch posture: part I (Figure 10)

Step 1: While sitting in the starting position, move the left leg away from the right.
Step 2: Bend the right leg and move the right foot so that the sole rests against the left thigh.
Step 3: Bend your left leg and gently move the left foot in front of your body.
Step 4: Take your left hand and bring it on the right side of your left foot. Now hold on to the left heel with the palm of the left hand and raise the foot so that it is in front of your forehead.
Step 5: Use your right hand to support the top of your left foot so that inside ankle of the left foot faces your forehead.
Step 6: Keep your back, neck and head erect. Stay in this position for 30 seconds.

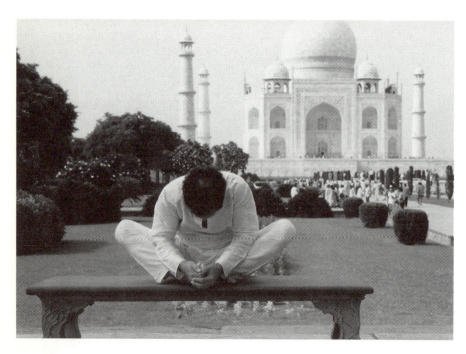

5 Legs, arms and back stretch posture

Leg and back stretch posture: part II (Figure 11)

Step 1: While sitting in the starting position, move the right leg away from the left.

Step 2: Bend the left leg and move the left foot so that the sole rests against the right thigh.

Step 3: Bend your right leg and gently move the right foot in front of your body.

Step 4: Take your right hand and bring it on the left side of your right foot. Now hold on to the right heel with the palm of the right hand and raise the foot so that it is in front of your forehead.

Step 5: Use your left hand to support the top of your right foot so that the inside ankle of the right foot faces your forehead.

Step 6: Keep your back, neck and head erect. Stay in this position for 30 seconds.

Posture 6

The candle and the plough: part I (Figure 12)

Step 1: Lie on your back. Let your hands rest by the side of your body. Without bending your legs, raise them 30 cm above the ground.

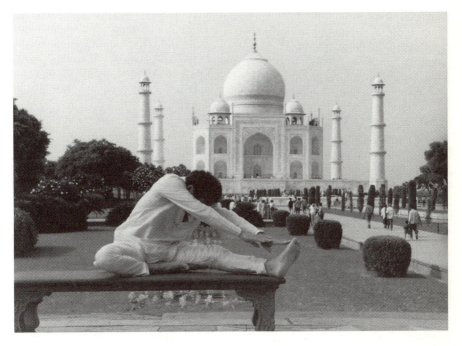

6 Arms and back stretch posture: part I

Step 2: Hold them there for 30 seconds and then lower them.
Step 3: Relax by breathing in and out. It should feel very good.

The candle and the plough: part II (Figures 13, 14, 15 and 16)

Step 1: Lie on your back. Let your hands rest by the side of your body. Without bending your legs, raise them 30 cm above the ground. Keep them in this position for 15 seconds and then raise them to a 45-degree angle (Figure 13). Hold them there for 15 seconds.
Step 2: Raise the legs to a 90-degree angle and stay there for 15 seconds (Figure 14).
Step 3: Put both hands on your waist and support your hips as you raise your body on your shoulders. Keep your hips in and heels out so that your shoulders, hips and heels make a straight line (Figure 15).
Step 4: Bring your legs behind your head so that your feet touch the ground. Hold your feet with your hands. Stay in this position for 15 seconds (Figure 16).
Step 5: Come back and stand on your shoulders. While in this position, open your legs sideways. Stay in this position for 15 seconds.
Step 6: Now come down in reverse order by making brief stops at the 90-degree angle, the 45-degree angle and 30 cm above the ground. Bring your legs

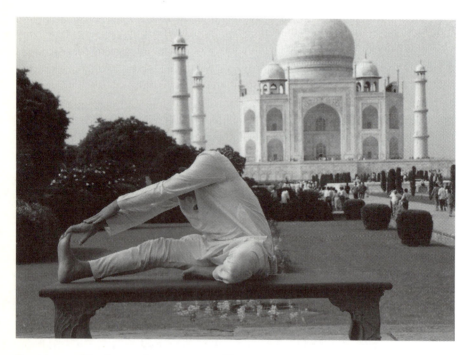

7 Arms and back stretch posture: part II

back to the original position. While breathing in and out observe the flow of your breathing. It should feel very good.

Posture 7

The bow posture (Figure 17)

Step 1: Lie on your stomach. Let your chin touch the ground.
Step 2: Bring your legs together and raise them while bending them at the knees.
Step 3: Hold your feet with your hands and raise your head. Now you are rolling on your belly button. Stay in this position for 30 seconds and then slowly come out of it. Relax by breathing in and out. Observe the flow of your breathing. It should feel very good.

Posture 8

The lotus posture: part I

Step 1: From the starting position, move your left leg at a distance from the right.
Step 2: Bend the right leg and move the right foot so that the sole sits next to the inside of the left thigh.

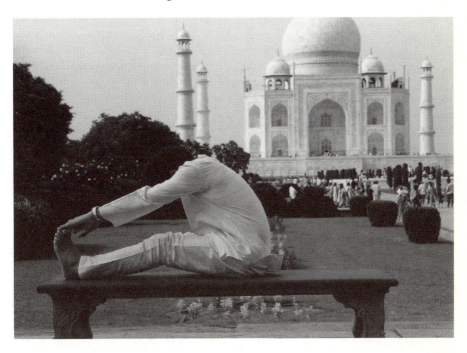

8 Arms and back stretch posture: part III

Step 3: Bend the left leg and place the left foot on the top of the right thigh, so that the heel touches the body.

Step 4: Your thumbs are touching your index fingers and your hands are resting on your knees. Keep your hips, back, neck and head erect. Your eyes are half or fully closed. While you inhale and exhale, observe the flow of your breathing. It should feel very good.

The lotus posture: part II

Step 1: From the starting position, move your right leg at a distance from the left.

Step 2: Bend the left leg and move the left foot so that the sole sits next to the inside of the right thigh.

Step 3: Bend the right leg and place the right foot on the top of the left thigh so that the heel touches the body.

Step 4: Your thumbs and index fingers are touching each other. Your hands are resting on your knees. Keep your hips, back, neck and head erect. Your eyes remain half or fully closed. While you inhale and exhale, observe the flow of your breathing. It should feel very good.

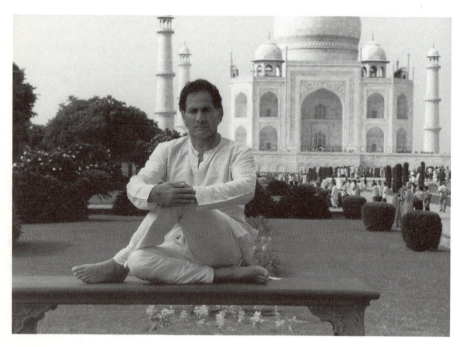

9 Student's posture: part I

The full lotus posture: part III (Figure 18) This position is a completion of the previous posture.

Step 1: While sitting in the previous half lotus posture, use your left hand to hold on to the left foot and remove the foot from beneath the right knee.

Step 2: When the left foot escapes the right knee, use your right hand to gently press down the right knee till it touches the ground.

Step 3: Now lift up the left foot and place it above the right thigh, so that the heel of the left foot touches the body.

Step 4: Your thumbs are touching your index fingers and your hands are resting on your knees. Keep your hips, back, neck and head erect. Your eyes remain half or fully closed. While you inhale and exhale, observe the flow of your breathing. It should feel very good.

Since the full lotus posture is most suitable for meditation, it is preferred over others. However, for the beginning student this position may be somewhat difficult at first. An easy posture which is a variation of the lotus position can be substituted.

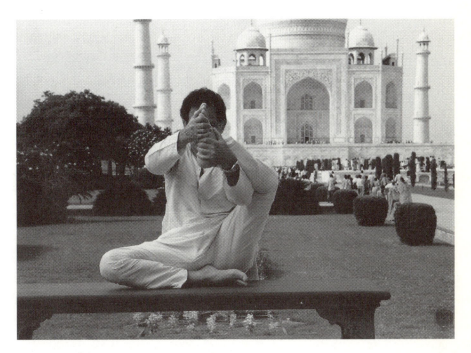

10 Leg and back stretch posture: part I

76   Yoga and Health

The lotus posture: part IV

The easy posture

Step 1:   Sit cross-legged.
Step 2:   Your thumbs are touching your index finger and your hands are resting on your knees.
Step 3:   Your eyes are half or fully closed. Your back, neck and head are erect. While breathing in and out, observe the flow of your breathing. It should feel very good.

Breathing exercises (*pranayama*)

Once you have perfected the easy or the lotus posture, you can do some simple breathing exercises. It is recommended that the breathing exercises should be done in a sitting position where the back is erect. For the beginner, the easy posture is most comfortable for these exercises.

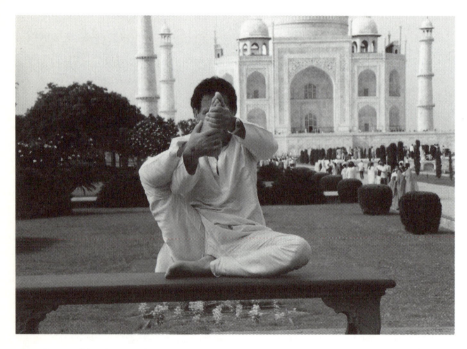

11   Leg and back stretch posture: part II

Exercise 1

Breathing through one nostril (count of 16-8-16): part I   Sit cross-legged. Keep your hips, back, neck and head erect.

Step 1: Take the middle three fingers of your right hand and put them on your forehead. Keep the thumb and the little finger free.
Step 2: Use the thumb to close the nostril nearest to it. Keep the other nostril open for breathing.
Step 3: From the open nostril breathe in for a count of sixteen.
Step 4: Retain the air in your lungs for a count of eight.
Step 5: Close the open nostril with the little finger. Open the other nostril by lifting the thumb.
Step 6: From the open nostril, breathe out for a count of sixteen. Do this exercise five times and then resume your normal breathing. Observe the flow of your breathing. It should feel very good.

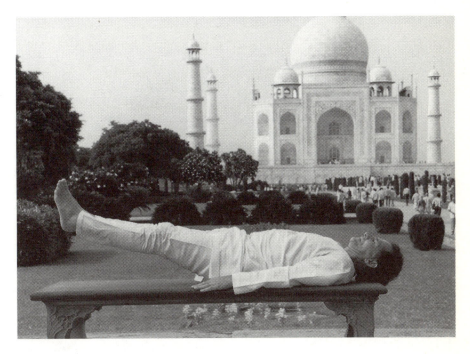

12   The candle and the plough: part I

78   Yoga and Health

Exercise 2

Breathing through one nostril (count of 16-8-8): part II   Sit cross-legged. Keep your hips, back, neck and head erect. (Note: this exercise is just like the previous one except that you breathe out for a count of eight instead of sixteen.)

Step 1:   Take the middle three fingers of your right hand and put them on your forehead. Keep the thumb and the little finger free.
Step 2:   Use the thumb to close the nostril nearest to it. Keep the other nostril open for breathing.
Step 3:   From the open nostril breathe in for a count of sixteen.
Step 4:   Retain the air in your lungs for a count of eight.
Step 5:   Close the open nostril with the little finger. Open the other nostril by lifting the thumb.
Step 6:   From the open nostril, breathe out for a count of eight. Do this exercise five times and then resume your normal breathing. Observe the flow of your breathing. It should feel very good.

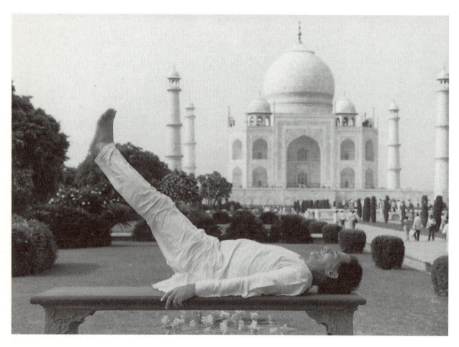

13   The candle and the plough: part II, step 1

Exercise 3

Breathing through one nostril and out through both Sit cross-legged or in the full lotus position. Keep your hips, back, neck and head erect.

Step 1: Take the middle three fingers of your right hand and put them on your forehead. Keep the thumb and the little finger free.
Step 2: Use the thumb to close the nostril nearest to it. Keep the other open for breathing.
Step 3: From the open nostril breathe in for a count of eight.
Step 4: Retain the air in your lungs for a count of eight.
Step 5: Open both nostrils and breathe out for a count of eight.

Do this exercise five times and then resume your normal breathing. Observe the flow of your breathing. It should feel very good.

Exercise 4

Fast inhalation and exhalation Sit cross-legged or in the full lotus position. Keep your hips, back, neck and head erect.

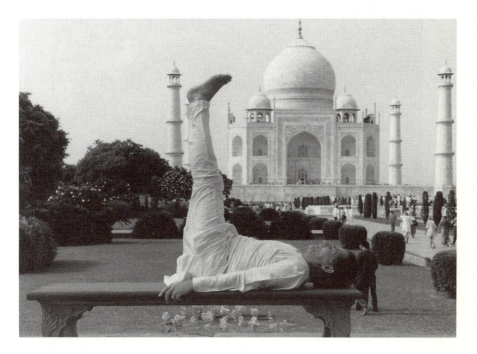

14 The candle and the plough: part II, step 2

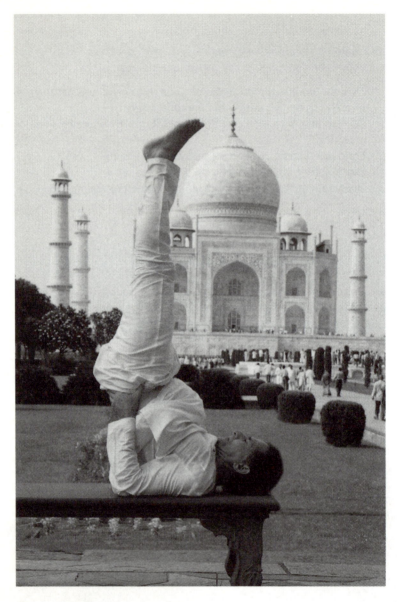

15 The candle and the plough: part II, step 3

Step 1: Take the middle three fingers of your left hand and put them on your forehead. Keep the thumb and the little finger free.
Step 2: Use the thumb to close the nostril nearest to it. Keep the other open for breathing.
Step 3: From the open nostril breathe in for a count of four.
Step 4: Open both the nostrils and breathe out for a count of four.

This exercise requires fast inhalation and exhalation. Do this exercise five times and then resume your normal breathing. Observe the flow of your breathing. It should feel very good.

Exercise 5

Breathing with the sound Aum   Sit in the easy or the lotus posture. Inhale as much air as you can so as to fill the lungs completely. Then exhale all the air. Perform this procedure twice. This will prepare the lungs for the next exercise, which uses the sound *Aum*.

Step 1: Breathe slowly to fill your lungs to their maximum capacity.
Step 2: Open your mouth completely and start uttering the sound *Aum* loudly.

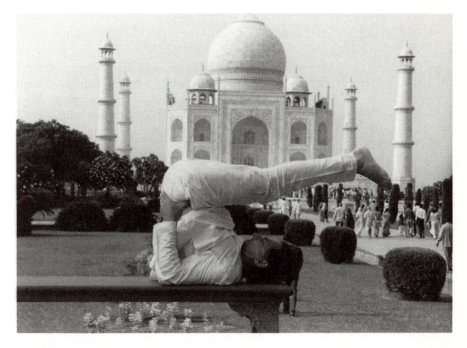

16   The candle and the plough: part II, step 4

82   *Yoga and Health*

Step 3:   When half the air is out, close your mouth but keep uttering the sound *Aum*. The sound, which vibrated outside before, will vibrate inside the body now. Keep saying the sound until you have no breath left.

Perform this exercise five times and then resume your normal breathing. Observe the flow of your breathing. It should feel very good.

Meditation exercises (*dhyana*)

Once you have perfected the breathing exercises, you can relax your body and calm the mind by adopting the dead man's posture. This position is a good preparation for the meditation exercises. In *Vibhutipada*, Patanjali describes meditation in terms of three stages of concentration ranging from the lowest to the highest. Meditation involves the spontaneous focusing of the mind on an object or an idea of one's choice. While attending to the object, the student might be distracted by the stimuli arising from external and internal sources. The goal is to bring back the mind to its chosen object despite these distractions. As the student perfects concentration, he can keep his mind on the object for a long time. By developing this mental skill, an individual can cleanse the mind of all distractions and thus becomes focused.

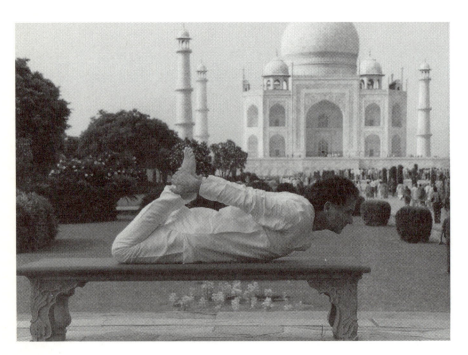

17   The bow posture

Exercise 1

Dead man's posture: part I Lie on your back. Let your arms rest next to your body. Close your eyes. Breathe in and out. Observe the flow of your breathing. It should feel very good.

Step 1:   Become aware of your toes. Tell yourself that there is no tension. They are fully relaxed.

Step 2:   Become aware of your feet. Tell yourself that there is no tension. They are fully relaxed.

Step 3:   Become aware of your ankles. Tell yourself that there is no tension. They are fully relaxed.

Step 4:   Become aware of your lower legs. Tell yourself that there is no tension. They are fully relaxed.

Step 5:   Become aware of your knees. Tell yourself that there is no tension. They are fully relaxed.

Step 6:   Become aware of your thighs. Tell yourself that there is no tension. They are fully relaxed.

Step 7:   Become aware of your hips. Tell yourself that there is no tension. They are fully relaxed.

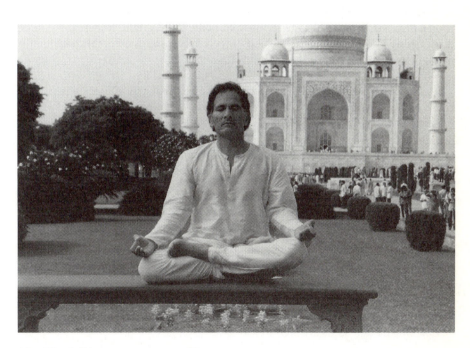

18   The full lotus posture: part III

Step 8: Become aware of your lower back. Tell yourself that there is no tension. It is fully relaxed.
Step 9: Become aware of your abdomen. Tell yourself that there is no tension. It is fully relaxed.
Step 10: Become aware of your upper back. Tell yourself that there is no tension. It is fully relaxed.
Step 11: Become aware of your chest. Tell yourself that there is no tension. It is fully relaxed.
Step 12: Become aware of your shoulders, arms, hands and fingers. Tell yourself that there is no tension. They are fully relaxed.
Step 13: Become aware of your neck and chin. Tell yourself that there is no tension. They are fully relaxed.
Step 14: Become aware of your lips and cheeks. Tell yourself that there is no tension. They are fully relaxed.
Step 15: Become aware of your eyes and forehead. Tell yourself that there is no tension. They are fully relaxed.

Now tell yourself that your entire body has no tension. It is fully relaxed. Stay in this position for one minute.

Dead man's posture: part II   This exercise is a continuation of the previous one. As you are in this relaxed position, tell yourself that you are looking at your body from a distance. You are just observing your body. It feels light. It feels weightless. It is floating in the air. It has no tension. It feels very good. Stay in this position for two minutes and enjoy the relaxation it brings.

Exercise 2

Meditation with the mantra so hum   Sit in the easy posture or the full lotus position. Bring thumb and index finger together. Place your hands on your knees. Keep your back, neck and head erect. Breathe in and out.

Step 1: As you breathe in, think about the sound *so*.
Step 2: As you breathe out, think about the sound *hum*.
Step 3: Keep your mind on *so hum*. If other ideas, emotions, feelings or sensations appear in your mind for attention, recognize them and then go back to the sound *so hum*. Do not be sidetracked by these distractions. Stay with the sound *so hum* for two minutes.

During the first few weeks of meditation with *so hum*, spend no more than two minutes on this exercise. After you have started feeling comfortable with the use of this sound, increase the time to three minutes. Other mantras which can be used to develop meditation skills are *hum so* and *Aum*.

Exercise 3

Meditation on a chosen object   Sit in the easy posture or the full lotus position. Bring thumb and index finger together. Place your hands on your knees. Your back, neck and head are erect. Keep your eyes closed. Breathe in and out.

Step 1:   Choose an image that has captivated you in the past. For example, it can be the image of the symbol *Aum* or the dancing *Shiva*. Keep the image as your focus.

Step 2:   If other ideas appear before your mind, recognize them but bring your attention back to the chosen image. Do not be sidetracked by these distractions.

Step 3:   Keep your mind on the chosen image for two minutes. As your concentration improves, there will be fewer distractions and you will be able to keep your mind on the chosen image for a longer duration.

Part IV
Yoga and Yoda

CHAPTER FOURTEEN

The *Star Wars* connection

Upon its release, George Lucas' fourth *Star Wars* film, *The Phantom Menace*, got mixed reviews. Some criticized it as misrepresenting Christian views, while others regarded it as 'spiritually hollow'. As a professor of philosophy and religion for thirty years, I became curious about the theological and ethical content of the *Star Wars* films. In order to probe deeper into the controversy, I watched all four films: *Star Wars: A New Hope*, *The Empire Strikes Back*, *Return of the Jedi* and *The Phantom Menace*. Moreover, I discussed the themes of the films with teenagers and adults who had been deeply touched by them. My personal impressions and conversations with others indicate to me that through these films, Lucas is making a genuine attempt to discover a common thread that links various religions of the world. He is interested in offering his vision of the spiritual life for the space age.

Though a number of ideas from the *Star Wars* films lend themselves to comparison with themes from Christianity, Judaism, Islam, Taoism and Zen, I will concentrate specifically on those raised in the *Yoga Sutras* and generally touched upon in the two major texts of Hinduism. On examining themes and the message of *Star Wars*, I realized that Lucas has been greatly influenced by the central ideas and mythology of Hinduism. His genius lies in his assimilation of the crucial ideas of the *Yoga Sutras*, the *Bhagavad Gita* and the epic *Ramayana*, and presenting them through the vehicle of *Star Wars*. As a filmmaker, Lucas is clearly a teacher with a 'thunderous voice'.

I will highlight a few important ideas which are shared by *Star Wars* and the Hindu texts mentioned above. The themes from *Star Wars* that can be compared to those of the *Yoga Sutras* and the Hindu epics are the essential nature of the Force; the unique student–teacher relationship; the lure of powers; *Prana* and Darth Vader's breathing; special talents of the Yogi and Yoda; psychological battle in the *Bhagavad Gita* and *Star Wars*; the conflict between good and evil; and similarities among the major players of the epic *Ramayana* and *Star Wars*.

A summary of the *Star Wars* films

Part I: Star Wars: A New Hope

In this film, Lucas raises and answers certain fundamental questions: What is the nature of the Force? How can it be used? How can it be abused? What is good? What is evil? Through the mouthpiece of Obi-Wan Kenobi, the great Jedi master, Lucas describes the nature of the Force, its use and abuse. Obi-Wan tells Luke

Skywalker that the Force is the underlying bonding principle of everything that exists. It is the glue that binds all things. The Force is the all-encompassing energy that works in human beings through their feelings and intuition. It is present in the tiniest cell and the largest galaxy. It possesses both dark and light sides. When one is training under the guidance of a Jedi master, one must complete the training without distractions from the lure of powers. Completed training helps the Jedi Knight to follow the light side of the Force. Those who are attracted by the powers acquired during training and are lured by the dark side of the Force may come to misuse the powers for personal gain and self-enhancement. Darth Vader is the embodiment of evil and the follower of the dark side. In contrast, Obi-Wan Kenobi represents the light side of the Force. He is training Luke Skywalker in the art of using the sabre through which he will experience and express the Force. At times, evil, as embodied by Darth Vader, looks so powerful that it is almost formidable. Though he had the potential to be a great Jedi Knight, Darth Vader turned to evil deeds. He represents the privation of good and expresses the dark side of the Force through anger, hatred, aggression, jealousy and violence. In contrast, Luke, who lacks such psychological blemishes as anger, fear, hatred and aggression, appears to be vulnerable. Luke is the follower of the light side and expresses it through compassion for others. He is fearless and is directed towards his goal of saving humanity from the destruction caused by Darth Vader and the evil Empire.

Part II: The Empire Strikes Back

The focus of this second *Star Wars* film is the training of the Jedi Knight under the tutelage of the master teacher, Yoda. Though Luke's training begins with Obi-Wan Kenobi in the first episode of *Star Wars*, it is Yoda who trains Luke in the ways of the Jedi Knights. Kenobi teaches Luke the art of using the sabre and offers him instructions on the utilization of feelings and intuition rather than intellect in experiencing the Force. When it comes to learning the difficult art of meditation and concentration, training takes place under the guidance of Yoda, the Jedi master.

Since Kenobi received his training from Yoda, he recommends Luke to do the same. Yoda is a highly accomplished Jedi who had trained Jedi Knights for 800 years. When he first meets Luke, Yoda is 900 years old. He puts Luke on a strict schedule of physical and psychological exercises. Luke's training consists of physical endurance through running, hanging upside down from a tree, moving stones from a distance, and the power of concentration. Through meditation, Luke learns to see the present, past and future, and people who are long gone.

Luke's training under Yoda takes place through an ideal student–teacher relationship. It is one-to-one training where Yoda is completely involved with Luke's total development. Yoda is gentle, observant and firm, and never gets upset. He teaches Luke through personal example. The Force is strong in Luke. In order to develop this Force and feel it, Yoda instructs Luke to get rid of anger and fear and to be patient, determined and a doer. Since anger, fear and hatred represent the dark side of the Force, Luke should eradicate them from his personality. Yoda offers three very important lessons during the training. First, both the dark and the light sides of the Force are within each person. When Luke fights Darth Vader, he will actually be fighting his own dark side. Second, the Force should always be used for benevolence, and never for attack. And third, a Jedi Knight does not try but does. Though Yoda is very small in stature, by using his power of concentration he shows Luke how to lift the starship from the marshy river.

Part III: Return of the Jedi

In this film, Luke arrives at the abode of Yoda to complete his training. Yoda informs him that there is nothing left that can be taught him by his teacher. To become a full Jedi Knight, Luke must undergo personal growth by going inward. He must delve into his own psyche to bring about the realization that both the dark and light sides of the Force are within him. Since his life is a clash of these two sides, he must fight the dark side and subdue it with the help of the light side. The dark side is clearly represented by his father, Darth Vader. Luke must fight him with all that he has learned from Obi-Wan Kenobi and Yoda. Only when Luke confronts Darth Vader in person and defeats him will he complete his training and thus become a Jedi Knight.

Luke, who senses the existence of some goodness in Darth Vader, tries to tap into it by convincing the latter to renounce his evil ways. The two of them fight and Luke defeats Darth Vader. When the evil Emperor tries to kill Luke, Darth Vader performs a fatherly act by eliminating the Emperor and thus saving his son's life. As a father, Darth Vader removes his mask so that he can see his son with his own two eyes. The mask symbolizes life for him and death for others. Once it is removed Darth Vader dies. But before he does so, he is able to express the light side of the Force by showing compassion for his son. Luke performs the last rites by cremating his father's body to purify it of all its evil deeds. In the last scene, when victory is being celebrated, Darth Vader as Anakin Skywalker is seen with the spirits of Obi-Wan Kenobi and Yoda. This is a reminder that Jedis do not die, they become one with the Force and are available for guidance to future generations. This completes Luke's training as a Jedi Knight because he has won victory over the dark side that resides within him.

The Yoga system

Yoga presents an artistically crafted picture of a human being including both psychophysical and spiritual aspects. The psychophysical part, consisting of the body, senses and mind, is a changing vehicle used by the true self, which is the unchanging spiritual force residing at the core of each human being. The entire cosmos is an expression of the infinite consciousness, which is the life force within everything. Though we appear to be separate individuals operating within our own tiny universes, we are all connected through this infinite force. Boundless and all-encompassing, this infinite conscious force is the glue that keeps everything together. It is present in all of us and we are connected to it as centres to a circle. The hub of this infinite consciousness lies in the human heart in the form of an unchanging spiritual force. The psychophysical self as a conglomeration of the body, senses and mind acts as a radio that transmits the waves of this cosmic force. If the vehicle of the psychophysical self is poorly constructed, it will not be able to send forth the spiritual signal of the force in its pure form. In order to make the psychophysical self, the perfect vehicle for the expression of the spiritual force, Yoga offers a step-by-step procedure. The mastery of the body, senses and the mind takes place in the ideal educational environment involving a special student–teacher relationship under the proper guidance of an accomplished Yoga teacher.

The method of training the student consists of eight steps which aim to perfect the entire person. The first step offers non-violence, non-lying, non-stealing, non-craving and non-possessiveness as five moral principles to prepare the body and the mind for the arduous inward journey. The second step embraces five disciplines of purity, contentment, austerity, self-study and ego-surrender as positive principles of physical and mental hygiene. These ten rules of physical and mental control help the student become fully focused so as to undertake the difficult task of the purification of the entire person.

The next two steps involve an elaborate array of physical and breathing exercises. Yoga emphasizes 64,000 physical postures which are designed to make every part of the body disease-free and ageless. Since a number of these postures imitate the way various animals, birds and insects relax, by mastering them the Yoga student gains knowledge of the nature of these creatures.

The next step of breathing control is crucial to the training of a Yoga student. Breathing is regarded as the vehicle through which the life force (*prana*) is captured from the outside and transmitted to the lungs and the heart. The heart distributes this force to various parts of the body and the brain. Through breathing exercises, the student learns voluntary control of inhalation, retention and exhalation, and is able to regulate the intake of the life force (*prana*). When the lungs and the heart are cleansed through the exercises, the student is able to develop full control of emotions of anger, fear, hatred, aggression, joy, delight and exhilaration.

The next four steps make up the meditative stage. In the first one, the student is trained to control the sense organs by cutting off the contact between them and their objects. Here one learns to withdraw consciousness from the sense organs and though the organs remain open, they stop performing their usual functions. By controlling the influence of the external world, the student is now prepared for the next three steps of concentration. Here one takes the inward journey by concentrating on various levels of consciousness. Through the perfection of these meditative steps, the accomplished student gets in touch with the underlying spiritual source residing at the core of his being.

By mastering the eight steps of the Yoga method, the student's body, senses and mind are transformed into a perfect vehicle through which the infinite cosmic force expresses itself uninterruptedly. This spontaneous flow of the force bestows the individual with extraordinary powers. Examples of some of these powers are levitation, knowledge of the past, present, future, other minds and the language of birds and animals as well as seeing things from far away, flying through space, moving objects from a distance and developing control of hunger and thirst. However, Yoga teachers constantly caution trainees and accomplished students not to be lured by these powers because they will mislead them to unacceptable ends. Since attachment to these powers impedes spiritual growth, the Yoga masters strongly recommend transcending them so that the student progresses towards the achievement of oneness with the infinite cosmic force.

A comparison of *Star Wars* and the Yoga method

The Force

What is the nature of reality? This is one of the major questions in the history of science, philosophy and religion. Answers to it have resulted in attempts to uncover the unity that underlies the diversity of existence. Depending upon one's discipline, this unitary principle has been variously designated as matter, mind, spirit or consciousness. Concerned with the mystery of human existence, the Yoga system describes the nature of reality by using the term 'consciousness', which is general enough to bring together the disciplines of science, philosophy and religion, and sufficiently specific to be applicable to the human reality. In the Yoga terminology, consciousness is perceived both as infinite and finite. As infinite, consciousness is all-encompassing reality that is present in everything. In its boundless aspect, infinite consciousness supports the universe and everything in it. Moreover, in its concrete expression, consciousness is present as the life force in every living being. In human beings it is called the spiritual force or consciousness. The relationship of the infinite and the finite consciousness can be compared to that of a circle to its centre. The cosmic consciousness is like an infinite circle whereas all manifested things are the centres through which this consciousness expresses itself concretely. There is nothing in the cosmos that is not connected by consciousness. It is present in the tiniest cell and the largest galaxy and is the glue that binds everything in the universe.

In a similar way to the Yoga system, George Lucas is interested in finding a common term that will be equally acceptable to science, philosophy and religion. To avoid controversies associated with terms such as 'consciousness', 'energy' and 'spirit', he uses the neutral term 'Force', which while capturing the essential shades of meaning associated with the other terms, stays clear of their ambiguity.

The Force is all-encompassing energy that surrounds us and binds everything together. One can also feel the Force around and within oneself because it expresses itself in the tiniest cell and the largest galaxy. As energy, it injects life into everything and is the glue that keeps all existence bound together.

The Force possesses both light and dark sides. These two are present in everything including human beings. When one gives in to the dark side, one performs evil deeds through which one brings harm to oneself and others. The dark side is displayed through anger, fear, hatred, deviousness and aggression. One who follows the light side executes good actions through which one saves oneself and others. Lack of anger, fear, hatred, deviousness and aggression are the hallmark of the followers of the light side. The goal is to develop the light side of the Force and to express it in deeds throughout one's life.

The rigorous training of the Jedi Knights highlights the development and the expression of the Force in their daily lives. Luke Skywalker, Obi-Wan Kenobi and Yoda are examples of those whose lives are dedicated to the expression of the light side of the Force; the evil Emperor, Darth Vader and his supporters follow the dark side of the Force and are driven to destruction and control of the universe. Yoda as the Jedi master par excellence is capable of experiencing the Force without distortion. Through perfecting the art of meditation and by forming an intimate relationship with nature, Yoda has gone farther than any of his Jedi students in the knowledge and use of the Force. So finely tuned are his intuitive faculties that Yoda is capable of experiencing the Force directly. In contrast, the evil Emperor and Darth Vader are examples of those who have turned to the dark side of the Force and though they appear to be invincible, the Jedi Knights are skilful in destroying these formidable opponents.

Method and the student–teacher relationship

To tap the spiritual force residing within, Yoga offers an eightfold method. Through a step-by-step procedure, the teacher of Yoga guides the student in the learning of good habits of the body, heart and mind. Since the goal is the perfection of the entire person, the student undertakes an austere training by adopting certain moral rules and principles of personal hygiene, by following a strict routine of physical and breathing exercises, and by practising the difficult discipline of meditation. All this is done under the guidance of a Yoga master.

Like other Indian systems, Yoga follows an ancient educational tradition involving a special teacher–disciple relationship. In the Sanskrit language, a teacher is called a guru, one who takes the student from darkness to light. Since the focus of the Yoga training is to realize the infinite conscious force that resides within the person, the guru–student relationship is of paramount importance. A guru is a multi-dimensional person who is a full-time teacher, a master of the art, a spiritual mentor and a fatherly figure. When a guru accepts a student, he forms a lifelong relationship with him and imparts to him all of his knowledge. Because of this special rapport and commitment, a student is carefully chosen. To be trained in the Yoga method, the student must show to the guru that he is capable of learning as well as worthy of knowledge. Humility and commitment are the two fundamental principles followed by the student. Humility lies in the surrendering of the lower mind to the higher self, which involves letting go of one's previous learning for the sake of the knowledge of the inner force. Commitment requires learning the steps of the method with a focused mind and practising it with a fanatic zeal and full concentration until one's goal of self-realization is reached.

The education of Jedi Knights is similar in some ways to the schooling of Yoga students. Before an individual can be trained as a Jedi Knight, he must reveal the strength of the Force within him. Since both Luke Skywalker and his father, Anakin Skywalker, demonstrate the strong presence of the Force within them, Obi-Wan Kenobi and Yoda accept them as trainees. Once Luke is selected, in a similar way to his Yoga counterpart, he undertakes rigorous physical and psychological training to gain complete control of his body, senses and mind.

Furthermore, Luke's education involves understanding and moving beyond anger, hatred, aggression, deviousness, egoism and impatience. Since these psychological blemishes hinder a Jedi's progress towards the experience of the Force, they must be transcended. In contrast, his father, Anakin Skywalker, gives in to anger, hatred, aggression and deviousness and ends up becoming Darth Vader, the embodiment of the dark side of the Force.

During Luke's training in meditation, Yoda acts as a perfect guru who is totally involved in the education of his disciple. When Yoda puts Luke on a strict schedule of rigorous physical and psychological exercises, he acts as his teacher, spiritual mentor and father. Furthermore, Yoda trains Luke by remaining calm, observant, firm, helpful and deeply involved in the spiritual growth of his student. Once, during a difficult part of his training when Luke feels frustrated because he is unable to lift the starship from the marshy water, Yoda provides a demonstration that is simultaneously an inspiration. Though tiny in size, Yoda miraculously lifts the starship by the movement of a single finger.

Like the Yoga teachers, both Obi-Wan Kenobi and Yoda teach Luke other important skills that are essential for a Jedi Knight. These include the art of unlearning what one has learned through the senses as well as relearning the art of feeling the Force without thinking.

The lure of powers

The rigorous training of the Jedi Knights, which is similar to the schooling of a Yoga student, gives rise to many unusual powers. Through the mastery of the body, senses and mind, the Jedi Knight gains access to the ways of the Force. This leads to the development of powers of levitation, flying through space, moving objects from a distance, mimicking the call of a bird or an animal, healing others and slowing the ageing process. Moreover, an accomplished Jedi develops the power of knowing the present, the past and the future.

In the Yoga system, students are given a stern warning not to be lured by these unusual powers because they will impede their progress towards spiritual realization. Those who give in to these powers become egotistical and might employ them to hurt others and themselves. While others use the same powers to heal and comfort those who are undergoing pain and suffering.

In *Star Wars*, one of the central themes is a clash between the use of the dark side and the light side of the Force. Since the Force is neutral energy, a trained Jedi is free to use it either negatively or positively. During the training of Jedi Knights, both Obi-Wan Kenobi and Yoda caution them to beware of lure of the dark side of the Force. Darth Vader, a trained Jedi who is enticed by the dark side of the Force, employs his unusual powers through such deeds as controlling the kingdom by devious means, and attacking and inflicting pain on innocent people. He is evil and the embodiment of anger, hate, fear and aggression. He fights for selfish gain by foul means. In contrast, Luke Skywalker is a good Jedi Knight who employs the light side of the Force by displaying it through fearlessness and benevolence. During one of his training sessions, Luke is told by Yoda that he should use the Force for knowledge and not for attack, and should never strike in anger. Though Luke hears this advice, he fails to put it into practice. In one of the sabre fights with Darth Vader, Luke strikes him in anger and pays the dear price of losing his hand. Similarly, in the first *Star Wars* film, Obi-Wan Kenobi warns Darth Vader that if he strikes him down in anger, Obi-Wan will become stronger and unbeatable, and he does. Through these two episodes, the *Star Wars* films emphasize the importance of controlling anger. When an action is done in anger the power of the light side of the Force is depleted in the doer and at the same time it is enhanced in the object acted upon. Since anger and hatred are impediments to the realization of the light side of the force, they should be subdued. With complete mastery over anger, a good Jedi Knight fights evil without seeking any reward. To fight evil and eradicate it is the fulfilment of a Jedi Knight's duty.

The breathing of Darth Vader and prana of Yoga

There are points of similarity between the forced breathing of Darth Vader and the Yoga view of *prana*. Darth Vader is Anakin Skywalker seduced by the dark side of the Force. By turning to the dark side, Darth Vader becomes evil and an angel of death. In his long, black robe and breathing mask, he appears to be more like a machine than a human being. Since he cannot depend upon his own flawed breathing apparatus he needs the help of his breathing mask. Without the mask he would die. Darth Vader's forced breathing is a symbol of death. By turning to the dark side of the Force, he has also turned away from life. His forced breathing through the mask is a fall from the grace of life and the light side of the Force. Throughout his life, Darth Vader is driven to doing evil deeds, which hurt and inflict pain on others. Only at the end does he turn to the light side of the Force by performing a good act that saves Luke's life at the hands of the evil Emperor. Though he knows that he will surely die without the breathing mask, he takes it off to see his son's face with his own eyes. This compassionate fatherly act costs Darth Vader his evil life but it also unites him with such great spirits as Obi-Wan Kenobi and Yoda.

The Yoga system also assigns a special place to breathing. *Pranayama*, which is one of the eight steps of the Yoga method, discusses the importance of breathing in detail. In Sanskrit, the terms *prana* and *yama* mean 'life force' and 'control'. Putting the two together, *pranayama* refers to the control of life force. The act of breathing is the vehicle through which the life force (*prana*) is captured from the outside. Through the lungs, it is transmitted to the heart which in turn distributes it to all parts of the body. As the life force, *prana* comes very close to the idea of the Force in *Star Wars*. It is through the force of *prana* that human beings are alive and connected to the rest of the universe. When this life force *(prana)* is properly trained and used, it can lead the individual to perform acts of compassion thereby enhancing one's life, as well as those of other human beings. However, when improperly employed by an individual, it can turn him into a tyrant who can inflict pain and suffering on others. The correct use of the life force makes life possible by connecting us to others, whereas incorrect employment of the force separates us from others.

Yoga and Yoda

An ideal Yoga teacher and a model Jedi master are similar in some respects. The true Yoga teacher is called a Yogi, one who by mastering the physical, breathing and meditation exercises has gained access to the spiritual force. His abode is in the calmness of a forest where he has retreated to a solitary place, and lives alone without any material possessions. He has developed the qualities of detachment from objects of senses, rewards of actions and attraction to desires. When a Yogi sees that a student has prepared himself and made himself worthy of his teachings, he accepts him as his pupil.

Training in the difficult art of Yoga begins in an ideal educational environment where the Yogi is fully involved in the total development of the disciple, acting as his teacher, spiritual mentor and father, and guiding him to the realization of the spiritual force within. Similarly, when Luke Skywalker goes to further his education with Yoda, he finds the latter living alone in a cave in the calmness of a forest on a remote island unspoiled by the artifacts of civilization. Yoda is a perfect example of a Jedi master who, by developing an empathetic closeness to nature and through the continuous practice of meditation, has fully trained himself in the ways of the Force. Yoda is also an experienced teacher because he has trained Jedi Knights for at least 800 years. On observing the strong presence of the Force in Luke and his high motivation to become a Jedi Knight, Yoda accepts him as his pupil and teaches him all that he knows. By continuously practising meditation on a daily basis, similar to a Yogi, Yoda has developed many unusual abilities, which set him apart from ordinary people. These are the powers of levitation, moving objects from a distance, knowing the past, present and future, mimicking the call of animals, healing others and defying the ageing process. Both the Yogi and Yoda teach their pupils the proper use of these powers, which is to help humanity. All in all, both the Yogi and Yoda are ideal gurus who act as superb teachers of physical and psychological skills, and who by providing the spiritual focus guide their pupils to the realization of the Force within.

The Bhagavad Gita *and* Star Wars *(psychological battle)*

In the Indian philosophical tradition, the Yoga system of Patanjali and the *Bhagavad Gita* are closely connected. The *Bhagavad Gita*, which is a religious-philosophical text, accepts the major points of the Yoga system and applies them to the training of a royal warrior. It opens with a description of a war to be fought between two royal families related by blood. Arjuna and his four brothers represent the good side whereas his one hundred cousins symbolize the evil side. Though Arjuna and his cousins receive comparable training from the same teachers, the cousins are lured by anger, hate, deviousness and aggression, and turn to evil by stealing the kingdom by unrighteous means. Before the battle to win back the kingdom from the evil cousins starts, Arjuna glances at the warriors and sees brothers, relatives and teachers on both sides. In spite of the fact that his cousins are evil, he cannot justify killing them. He gets confused and refuses to fight. Krishna, who is Arjuna's charioteer and teacher, makes him aware of the spiritual force within, and directs him to fight evil even when it is represented by his own blood relatives. Krishna compares Arjuna's righteous battle with his cousins to a struggle within his own mind. Though Arjuna has been educated as a warrior by the best teachers, his training is not yet complete because he lacks the knowledge, determination and one-pointed attention to fight the psychological battle raging within. After a long discourse, Krishna convinces Arjuna with the truth that the real battle is between the good and evil tendencies within his own psyche. By defeating his cousins in the battlefield, Arjuna will win not only the war but also a great victory over his divided psyche and thus will raise himself to the rank of an ideal warrior.

In the *Star Wars* films, a similar battle is raging between the evil symbolized by Darth Vader and the good represented by the rebel forces of Luke Skywalker. The evil Emperor and Darth Vader control the Empire by devious means and want to crush the rebellion. The evil forces of Darth Vader are large and invincible whereas the good forces of Luke are small and vulnerable. Darth Vader has the death star and all the advantages of a space age army and technology. In contrast, the rebel forces consist of a strange team of Luke Skywalker, Han Solo, Chewbacca, the Droid (CP30) and R2D2.

Like the battle in the *Bhagavad Gita,* the stage is set for a war between what appears to be a large and undefeatable army of the evil forces of Darth Vader and a small vulnerable army of the good forces of Luke Skywalker. Similar to Krishna who advises Arjuna to fight the war against his own evil cousins by convincing him that the battle is actually being fought within his own psyche, Yoda tells Luke Skywalker that Darth Vader, the embodiment of evil, is Luke's real father. During his training under Obi-Wan Kenobi, Anakin Skywalker learns a great deal. When he is seduced by the power of the dark side of the Force, he quits before completing his education and becomes Darth Vader, the embodiment of evil. Yoda informs Luke that both the dark and light sides of the Force reside within each person. The dark side within him is his father. When Luke fights Darth Vader, he will be battling with the dark side of his own self. By winning his battle against Darth Vader, he will win the spiritual battle within his own psyche. This victory of the light side over the dark side of the Force will assure him the status of a Jedi master. When Luke is encouraged by Yoda, he goes on to fight his evil father and defeats him in battle. This victory over Darth Vader integrates Luke's psyche as well as making him a full Jedi Knight.

The epic Ramayana *and* Star Wars

While watching the four parts of the *Star Wars* films, I also observed similarities with some crucial themes as portrayed in the Indian epic *Ramayana*. Central to the epic is the battle between good and evil. King Ravana of Sri Lanka, his brother, his son and his huge army of demons, which represent the forces of evil, plan to conquer the entire universe. Frightened by Ravana's devious plan, gods approach the preserver of the universe, Vishnu, and request him to come down to the earth to save it from destruction. Vishnu consents to this plan and takes the human form of Rama, the prince of Ayodhya. Ravana's exploits make him so fearless that he arrives at the abode of Rama and kidnaps the latter's wife Sita and keeps her as his prisoner in Sri Lanka. Rama, the great warrior, assisted by his brother Lakshmana, the king of serpents, accompanied by Hanuman, the king of the monkeys, helped by Null-Neel, the pair of engineers, and guided by Geedhraj, the king of birds, battles against the invincible armies of the evil Ravana. The war between the two sides is fought with the help of space age weapons. Ravana, his brother, his son and his generals are trained warriors who have been lured by the dark side of the force. They abuse this power by inflicting pain on innocent people. In order to defeat Ravana's invincible power of the dark side, even Prince Rama, the god-incarnate, needs the help of Lakshmana, Hanuman, the Null-Neel pair and the all-knowing Geedhraj. Only when the best among humans, monkeys, animals and birds, representing the good forces of the earth, come together are they able to defeat the undefeatable armies of Ravana and put an end to his evil empire.

The story and characters of *Star Wars* appear to be similar to those of the epic *Ramayana*. The evil Emperor, Darth Vader and their space age armies, representing the dark side of the Force, are like the evil Ravana, his son and his ferocious army of demons. Though Darth Vader in *Star Wars* presents himself as a formidable opponent, he is beaten by the combined efforts of Luke Skywalker, Han Solo, Chewbacca, R2D2, the Droid (CP30) and Yoda. Similarly, in *Ramayana*, Prince

Rama, the emotional Lakshmana, the monkey king, Hanuman, the engineer pair Null-Neel and the knowledgeable Geedhraj defeat the invincible armies of Ravana. The parallels between the characters of Prince Rama and Luke Skywalker, emotional Han Solo and feisty Lakshmana, the strong Chewbacca and the fearless monkey Hanuman, the technological wonder pair of CP30-R2D2, and the inseparable twin engineers Null-Neel, and the all-knowing Yoda and the knowledgeable Geedhraj are striking. Furthermore, in *Star Wars*, after the destruction of the evil empire of Darth Vader, the kidnapped Princess Leia is returned to her kingdom, and as the victory is being celebrated with great pomp and show, it is blessed by the spirits of Anakin Skywalker, Obi-Wan Kenobi and Yoda. Similarly in the epic *Ramayana*, after the armies of King Ravana are defeated, Princess Sita is returned to her kingdom in Ayodhya and a huge victory celebration takes place which is blessed by the gods and the departed soul of Rama's father.

CHAPTER FIFTEEN

Conclusions

I have written *An Introduction to Yoga Philosophy* to reveal Yoga's appeal at the scholarly, scientific, practical, personal and popular levels. The first two parts address the needs of scholars and students whose interest lies in the theoretical aspects of Yoga. The third part dealing with Yoga's connection to health, healing and wholeness is directed at the general reader whose interests are practical in nature. At present there are close to 10 million Americans practising some form of Yoga involving physical exercises for improving bodily health, or breathing exercises for cultivating emotional control, or meditation exercises for gaining spiritual strength. The number of Yoga practitioners worldwide is also growing. What appeals to people at the grassroots level is Yoga's view of the whole person in possession of total physical, psychological and spiritual health. This is an intriguing model for the medical and humanistic sciences to imbibe during the twenty-first century and the new millennium. I have added the fourth part of the text to show that the major practical and spiritual themes of Yoga, which have enchanted human beings from all strata of society during its 2,500 year long history, are still inspirational for the likes of George Lucas in the twentieth century. Through the *Star Wars* films, where he presents his version of spirituality for the technological age, Lucas makes liberal use of some of the essential elements of the Yoga philosophy and themes from the Hindu epics. The incorporation of the central issues of Yoga into the *Star Wars* films is a clear indication that Yoga is going to be with us for a long time. This is certainly good news for seekers of spiritual health and wholeness who would be delighted to see Yoga become the favourite of humanity during the new century and the new millennium.

Glossary

Abhinivesha: clinging to life or intense fear of death. It is one of the five afflictions (*kleshas*).

Aesthetics: a branch of philosophy that deals with beauty as it manifests itself in nature and works of art.

Aham Brahman asmi: a mantra used in meditation, which means 'I am identical with Brahman, the ultimate reality'.

Ahamkara: ego sense. It is the principle of individuation that produces the sense of I, me, my and mine. In the Samkhya philosophy, it is the second evolute of material reality.

Antarangas: the three internal steps of meditation in the Yoga method.

Asamprajnata: a state of meditation or trance, which transcends all objects.

Asanas: various physical postures involved in the Yoga practice.

Ascetic: an individual who withdraws from the world and devotes one's life to meditative practices.

Ashtanga: the major method of Yoga meant for the serious student. It consists of eight steps involving both physical and meditation exercises, which will help the student reach enlightenment.

Asmita: egoism. It is one of the five afflictions (*kleshas*) through which one ignorantly identifies the real self with the psychophysical self.

Atman: the inner self or the divine spark that resides at the core of a person's being.

Aum: the mystical symbol *Om*, which is the highest mantra. All the sounds of the world have their source in it.

Avidya: ignorance, one of the afflictions that prevents a person from reaching enlightenment or omniscience.

Ayurveda: one of the Hindu scriptures that deals with health and healing.

Bhagavad Gita: literally, 'The Song of God'. The text of the *Bhagavad Gita* constitutes one of the eighteen chapters of the Mahabharata.

Bhakti Yoga: the path of devotion. One of the three paths by which one may attain illumination.

Brahma: the god who resides at the head of the Hindu trinity, and is considered the creator of the universe.

Brahman: the ultimate reality or the objective universal self in contrast to Atman, which is the subjective self in each human being.

Buddhi: the principle of cosmic intelligence. It is the finest product of *prakriti*. At an individual level, it is the source of all inspiration, whereas at the cosmic level all creative endeavours flow from it. It is a place where illumination occurs.

Chitta: our ordinary mind or consciousness, which consists of the three cognitive functions of intelligence, ego-sense and understanding.
Cultic Yoga: the popularized form of Yoga brought to the West by numerous, self-appointed gurus, who prey upon the willingness of their followers to believe in a form of 'instant nirvana'.

Determinism: a philosophical doctrine that all objects and events are caused by some prior conditions independent of human will.
Dharana: the first meditative step of the Yoga method where concentration still involves distractions.
Dharma: righteousness. One of the four goals of life.
Dharma mega samadhi: the final contemplative state that showers virtue and merit.
Dhyana: the second meditative step of the Yoga method. It is the unbroken flow of consciousness towards an object.
Dvesha: repulsion. One of the five afflictions (*kleshas*).

Ekagrata parinama: contemplative consciousness that has moved from one-pointed to no-pointed concentration.
Ethics: a branch of philosophy that deals with moral values and principles.
Existential: pertaining to human existence or total interest in the human being and his destiny.
Existentialism: the school of philosophy developed by the philosopher Jean Paul Sartre that seeks to address the dilemmas of human life by denying most metaphysical explanations of existence and placing ultimate responsibility in the hands of the individual.

Gnana Yoga: the path of knowledge. This is the preferred path of philosophers, sages and thinkers.
Gunas: the three qualities that are the basic ingredients of the manifest universe.
Guru: a qualified spiritual teacher who has achieved enlightenment and can impart it to others.

Harvard Yoga: one of the four popularized forms of Yoga, celebrated by psychologists and clinical scientists, whose primary interest is the effects of meditation on various aspects of the human personality.
Himalayan Yoga: the true and authentic form of Yoga as practised in India since its inception. The term 'Himalayan' is applied to distinguish it from the other, popularized forms.
Hollywood Yoga: another popularized form of Yoga, deriving its name from the fact that its adherents have included many famous TV and film personalities. It depicts Yoga as nothing more than physical exercises that offer a slim body, restful sleep and a long life.

Indriyas: ten sense and motor organs.
Ishwara: the *Perfect Yogi* who can be used as an ideal to be pursued.

Kaivalya: the final goal of Yoga where an individual realizes the nature of the true self as pure consciousness. It also signifies total freedom from all limitations.
Kaivalyapada: the fourth and final part of the *Yoga Sutras*. It deals with the various layers of consciousness as well as the state of liberation.
Karma: action. It entails actions of the past lives whose effects determine our present existence on this earth.
Karma Yoga: one of the three paths whereby one may achieve illumination through action.
Katha Upanishads: one of the earliest philosophical texts of the Hindus.
Kleshas: the afflictions or hindrances of consciousness that prevent one from reaching enlightenment.
Krishna: the god-incarnate. Also the charioteer of Arjuna in the *Bhagavad Gita*.
Kriya Yoga: a preliminary path of Yoga for those who are not yet ready to devote themselves to the rigour of the higher practice.
Kurma nadi: a special kind of nerve, which has the shape of a tortoise. It resides in the region of the throat and controls anger, lust, pride, envy and infatuation. When a student of Yoga centres his mind on it, he gains control of his emotions.

Manas: the faculty of understanding that conceptualizes.
Mantra: a sacred sound-formula, which embodies within itself the secret of consciousness or reality.
Meditation: the practice of bringing the mind under control.

Neti neti: literally, 'Not this, not this'. This is one of the mantras used in meditation to caution the student that no descriptions of ultimate reality are adequate.
Nirbija: contemplation without a seed or fluctuation.
Nirodha: literally 'stoppage', 'extinction' or 'cessation'.
Nirodha parinama: contemplation where the mind is still involved in controlling distractions by focusing on a single idea.
Nirvicara: contemplation where one attains the super-reflective stillness. Here there is the dawning of utmost spiritual clarity.
Nirvitarka: contemplation where consciousness cleansed of all memory of its past contents achieves knowledge of the object directly.
Niyamas: the second step of the Ashtanga Yoga. It consists of five positive principles of cleanliness, contentment, austerity, self-study and self-surrender.

Pada: literally, 'chapter' or 'part'. Any one of the four parts of the *Yoga Sutras* text.
Patanjali: the founder of the Yoga system.
Philosophy: the science and discipline of thinking analytically. It involves an in-

depth analysis of fundamental concepts such as reality, truth, existence, freedom and the like.

Prakriti: in the Samkhya philosophy, the primal material reality or material nature. It consists of the three qualities (*gunas*). Through various combinations of these components different objects and creatures are formed in the universe.

Prakritic: pertaining to the created or manifest world.

Prana: the vital force of life, particularly as manifested in the breath.

Pranayama: the discipline of controlling and directing the vital force, usually through exercises that involve various patterns of regulating the breath.

Pratyahara: the fifth step of the Yoga method. Here one disconnects the sense organs from their objects.

Psychology: the science of studying and analysing the human mind, with an emphasis on various forms of cognition and emotional states.

Purusha: the conscious reality that experiences the universe. It is the spark of divinity in each human being.

Raga: one of the five afflictions (*kleshas*) that hinder the achievement of enlightenment. Raga means attachment.

Rajas: one of the three qualities (*gunas*). In particular, this is the principle of restless activity and passion.

Sabija: contemplation with seed involving a thought, image or object.

Sadhanapada: that part of the *Yoga Sutras* which deals with the method of Yoga practice.

Samadhi: trance, mental stillness or contemplation. It is also the eighth step of the Yoga method.

Samadhipada: that section of the *Yoga Sutras* which deals with the meaning and goal of Yoga as well as with attainment of trance or mental stillness.

Samkhya: the metaphysical philosophy forming the underpinnings and background of the Yoga system.

Samprajnata: the first kind of contemplation where the mind concentrates on reasoning, reflection, joy and ego-sense.

Samyama: one-pointed attention, formed from the workings of the three steps of concentration, meditation and absorption.

Sat chit ananda: infinite existence, awareness and joy. It is the ultimate goal of self-realization.

Sattva: one of the three ingredients of material reality. It is the quality of pure joy or good.

Savicara samadhi: the stage of contemplation where consciousness reflects on the nature of the ego-sense and how it constructs the principle of individuation and causes confusion between the real self and the ego self.

Savitarka samadhi: a stage of contemplation where consciousness reflects on the knowledge of the object by blending together word, meaning and content.

Science: the disciplined, analytical approach to understanding the world by means of observation, hypothesis and experimentation.
Self: the principle that experiences the world. It is referred to as 'I'.
Shiva: in the Hindu trinity, the god who is regarded as the Destroyer. However, it should be understood that this refers to destruction as the necessary prelude to renewed creation.
Sutra: literally, a 'thread'. It is a statement that 'threads' together a group of ideas for the purpose of brevity.

Tamas: one of the three ingredients of material reality. It is the principle of pure dullness or inertia.
Tat tvam asi: literally, 'You are that'. Your essence as a human being is identical with that of the universe.

Upanishads: the end parts of the Vedas. They are the earliest philosophical texts of the Hindus.

Vedas: the four ancient books on Hinduism. They contain the basic ideas of Hindu religion and philosophy.
Vibhuti: the accomplishments or special powers gained from disciplined Yoga practice. Though the *Yoga Sutras* outlines various such powers, the student is cautioned about their lure because they can act as hindrances to the achievement of the final goal of enlightenment.
Vibhutipada: the third part of the *Yoga Sutras* which deals with various steps of meditation and the accomplishments that can arise from the practice.
Vishnu: in Hinduism, the deity referred to as the Preserver. This deity, like *Shiva*, is often depicted as taking a distinct active interest in the affairs of human beings. According to the Hindu religion, *Vishnu* has taken various forms throughout history, appearing as Krishna, Rama, Buddha and even Jesus Christ.
Vritti: literally, 'modification'. When used in conjunction with the mind, it refers to modifications or fluctuations in the ordinary consciousness.

Yamas: restraints or controls. It is the first step of the Yoga method and involves five restraints of non-violence, non-lying, non-stealing, non-craving for sensual pleasure and non-possessiveness.
Yoga: literally, 'union'. The term refers to the system founded by Patanjali, offering a practical method for reaching union between the lower and the higher self. It also refers to disunion of oneself from the false view of reality.
Yoga Sutras: the foundational text of the Yoga system, which was compiled by Patanjali. It offers a simple and precise exposition of the various facets of the Yoga philosophy and practice.

Bibliography

Ajaya, Swami (1989) *Yoga Psychology*, Honesdale, Pa.: Himalayan Institute
Aranya, Swami Hariharamanda (1983) *Yoga Philosophy of Patanjali*, Albany, N.Y.: SUNY Press
Arya, Usharbudh (1974) *Superconscious Meditation*, Honesdale, Pa.: Himalayan Institute
Bilimoria, Purusottama (1974) *Yoga Meditation and the Guru*, New Delhi: Sterling Paperback
Chopra, Deepak (1993) *Ageless Body, Timeless Mind*, New York: Harmony Books
Feuerstein, George (1974) *The Essence of Yoga*, London: Rider & Company
Fields, Gregory P. (2001) 'Religious Therapeutics: Body and Health in Yoga and Ayurveda and Tantra', Albany, N.Y.: SUNY Press.
Iyengar, B.K.S. (1993) *Light on the Yogasutras of Patanjali*, San Francisco: HarperCollins
Malhotra, Ashok K. (1999) *Instant Nirvana*, New York: Oneonta Philosophy Studies
Malhotra, Ashok K. (1999) *Transcreation of the Bhagavad Gita*, Englewood Cliffs, N.J.: Prentice-Hall
Miller, Barbara Stoler (1998) *Yoga: Discipline of Freedom*, New York: Bantam Books
Mishra, Ramamurti (1987) *The Textbook of Yoga Psychology*, New York: Julian Press
Radha, S.S. (1978) *Kundalini Yoga for the West*, Boulder, Col.: Shambhala
Rama, Swami (1979) *Lectures on Yoga*, Honesdale, Pa.: Himalayan Institute
Singh, B.B. (n.d.) 'Translation of the Yogasutras', unpublished manuscript
Taimni, I.K. (1981) *The Science of Yoga*, Wheaton, Ill.: Theosophical Publishing House
Varenne, Jean (1976) *Yoga and the Hindu Tradition*, Chicago: University of Chicago Press
Wichler, Ian (1998) *The Integrity of the Yoga Darsana*, Albany, NY: SUNY Press

Index

abhinivesha 34–5
abhyasa 27
absorption, *see samadhi*
absorption transformation, *see ekagrata parinama*
afflictions, *see kleshas*
Aham Brahman asmi 13
ahamkara 7, 56; *see also* ego-sense
ananda 28
anger 96
animals, language of 45–6, 93, 98
arms and back stretch posture 67–8, 71–3
Arya, Usharbudh 15
asamprajnata samadhi 27–8, 32
asanas 9, 37–9, 64–5
ascetics 52
Ashtanga Yoga 8, 20, 33, 37, 64
asmita 28, 34–5
Aum sound 81–2, 84–5
austerity, *see tapas*
avidya 34–5
Ayurveda, the 18

Baba Ram Dass 52
Bhagavad Gita ix, 10, 35–6, 89, 98
Bhakti Yoga 11–12
bow posture 73, 82
Brahma 17
Brahman 13, 29
breathing 40, 62, 92, 96–7; *see also pranayama*
Buddha 52, 61
buddhi 7, 32, 50–1, 56
Buddhism 53

candle and plough 71–3, 77–81
charismatic leaders 16
chitta 7, 10, 12, 25, 33, 56
Christianity 53, 89; *see also* Jesus
clairvoyance 46
concentration 46, 92; *see also dharana*
consciousness
 contemplative 28, 31–2
 finite and infinite 93
 see also disturbances; fluctuations; pure consciousness

contemplative transformation, *see samadhi parinama*
cosmic force 62, 92–3
Cultic Yoga 15–16

dead man's posture 82–4
death
 fear of 34–5
 foreknowledge of 47
detached attitude 65
dharana 8–9, 20, 37, 42–3
dharma mega samadhi 57
dhyana 8–9, 20, 37, 42–3, 64, 82–5
disappearance of the body 47
disciplines 92; *see also niyama*
discriminative knowledge 6–7, 27, 37, 56–7
disturbances of consciousness 29–30, 63
drugs 52–3
dvesha 34–5
dynamic void 44

ego, the 53–4
ego-sense 32, 50–51, 56
egoism, *see asmita*
Einstein, Albert 30, 45
ekagrata parinama 43–4
empathy 46
The Empire Strikes Back 90–91
enlightenment 57

fire 48
fluctuations in the mind or consciousness 26–7, 31, 63; *see also chitta-vrittis*
flying, power of 49, 93, 95
the Force 93–9
friendship 47

Gandhi, Mahatma 39, 61
Gnana Yoga 7, 11, 14
gravity 49, 62
guna 10–11, 55
gurus 94

Hare Krishna movement 12, 53
Harvard Yoga 15
Hatha Yoga 15
healing 61–2

Himalayan Institute 40
Himalayan Yoga 15–16
Hinduism 17, 89
Hollywood Yoga 15
Huxley, Aldous 52

ignorance 36–7; *see also avidya*
indifference, *see tamasa*
individuation 32
intelligence, *see buddhi*
intuitive knowledge 31–2
Ishwara 29, 33–4

Jesus 52, 61

kaivalya 57
Kaivalyapada 19–21, 52
karma 35–6, 47, 54
Karma Yoga 11–12
King, Martin Luther 39
kleshas 33–5
kneeling posture 65–9
knowledge, sources of 26
Krishna 12, 53, 98
Kriya Yoga 20, 33–5

leg and back stretch posture 70, 75–6
levitation 48–9, 62, 93, 95, 97
life, clinging to, *see abhinivesha*
life force, *see prana*; *pranayama*
lotus posture 73–6, 83
Lucas, George 89, 93, 101

Maharishi Mahesh Yogi 53
manas 7, 56
mantras 12–13, 20, 29, 53, 84
master mediators 53–4
meditation ix, 8–10, 13, 15–16, 20, 29–30, 35, 37, 40, 42–3, 45, 49, 53, 63–4, 75, 82, 84–5, 90, 94–5, 97, 101
Mohammed the Prophet 52
moral restraints and principles 62, 92

Neti neti 13
Newton, Isaac 30, 45
nirbija 19, 28, 31–2, 42
nirodha 10, 25, 43
nirodha parinama 43–4
nirvicara 28
nirvicara samadhi 31
nirvitarka 28, 31–2

nirvitarka samadhi 31–2
niyamas 8–9, 37–9

objective reality, *see Prakriti*
Om sound-symbol 13, 29–30
one-pointed attention, *see samyama*
ordinary mind 55–7

pain, *see rajasa*
Patanjali 10–11, 16–19, 26–7, 29–30, 32–7, 39–44, 46–54, 57, 64, 81, 96
Perfect Yogi 29
personality 11–14
The Phantom Menace 89
philosophy ix, 3–4, 6, 10–11, 14, 17, 30, 61, 64, 87, 91, 99
pleasure, *see sattva*
posture 62, 65–76, 82–4, 92; *see also asana*
Prakriti 6–7, 31–2, 36–7, 44, 55–7
prana 40, 89, 92, 96–7
pranayama 8–9, 37–9, 49, 64, 76, 97
pratyahara 8–9, 37–41
psychics 46
psychology viii, 3–5, 10–14
pure consciousness 5–9, 11, 48, 50, 55, 61
Purusha 6–7, 31–7, 41, 48–51, 55–7

raga 34–5
rajasa 6–7, 10–12, 44, 55
Ramakrishna 52
Ramayana 89, 99–100
reasoning, *see vitarka*
reflection, *see vicara*
reincarnation 36, 46, 53
repulsion, *see dvesha*
restraint, *see yama*
restraint transformation, *see nirodha parinama*
Return of the Jedi 91

sabija 31–2
Sadhanapada 19–20, 33, 64
Sai Baba 52
samadhi 8–9, 19–20, 25, 27–8, 31–2, 37, 42–4, 48, 57
samadhi parinama 43–4
Samadhipada 19, 25
samana 48
Samkhya 6–7, 10–11, 14, 35–6, 55–6
samprajnata 27–8, 32
samyama 42–53

Sartre, Jean-Paul 52
Sat chit ananda 10, 13
sattva 7, 10–11, 13–14, 44, 55
savicara 28
savicara samadhi 31–2
savitarka 28
savitarka samadhi 31–2
science ix, 3–5, 8–9, 49, 61, 91, 99
seedless contemplation, *see nirbija samadhi*
self 3–4, 6–8, 11–13, 16, 19, 25–40, 42–3, 48–51, 55–7, 61–3, 89–90, 92, 96
sense-organ withdrawal, *see pratyahara*
Shiva 12, 17, 40, 84
siddhis 45
sleep 26
so hum sound 84
Star Wars 49–50, 89–90, 96–101
starting position 65–6
stillness of the mind 27–32; *see also samadhi*
student's posture 69–70, 74
supernormal powers 43–53, 95–6
sutra ix, 10, 19, 25–6, 29–30, 32, 37, 44–5, 50
svadhyaya 33–4
Swami Rama 53

tamasa 7, 10–12, 44, 55
*tapa*s 33, 53

Tat tvam asi 13
Mother Teresa 61
training in Yoga 92–7
tranquility
  higher levels of 31
  impediments to 29–30
Transcendental Meditation 13, 53
true self, *see Purusha*
truth bearing wisdom 31–2
Tutu, Desmond 39

udana 48–9, 62

vairagya 27
Vibhutipada 19–20, 42, 45, 82
vicara 28
violence and non-violence 39
Vishnu 17–18, 99
vital force, *see udana*
vitarka 28
vritti 10, 25

yamas 8–9, 37–9, 97
Yoga
  goal of 4, 8, 25–6, 33, 56, 63
  meaning of term 4, 25
  number of practitioners 99
Yogis 97–8

Zen 53

Mark Klingnell
"Husserl's Sense of Worlds"
The Philosophical Forum
Vol 31, #1 Spr 2000.